Advance Praise

This is a book that should have been written 100 years ago, before Dr Kellogg began his campaign of mutilating boys to keep them from masturbating. Lindsay Watson is exposing an issue that has been hidden for a century.

Anyone who has a male baby needs to be made acutely aware that there is NO need for circumcision and it has the potential to create life long problems for their child. Doctors need to refuse to participate in this mutilation. Hospitals and insurance companies should refuse to support or pay for circumcision. The easy question to ask any doctor, "Would you willingly cut off a part of your genitalia as an adult?" Most would not do this to themselves as adults willingly without compelling medical reasons. There is no reason for adults to do this to babies who cannot consent. Parents should never have the right to mutilate their child in the name of religion or tradition. If it is so important to a person's religion, they can choose to do it as an adult.

Read this book and learn how devastating this unnecessary practice is on the lives of men. Then let others know. Let's stop this barbaric and primitive practice.

Dr. Darrel Ray, **Ed.D.**, author of *Sex and God: How Religion Distorts Sexuality* and *The God Virus*.

24 February 2014

UNSPEAKABLE MUTILATIONS

CIRCUMCISED MEN SPEAK OUT

There can be no keener revelation of a society's soul than the way in which it treats its children. – Nelson Mandela

LINDSAY R. WATSON

Published by Lindsay R. Watson

Ashburton, New Zealand

Disclaimer: This book is informational only and should not be considered as a substitute for consulting a registered medical practitioner.

ISBN 13: 978-1495266577

ISBN 10: 1495266575

Editing: Lindsay Watson and Larry D. Wilson

Cover Art and Design: Alison Tieman

Illustrations: Chris Ebbert

Printed by CreateSpace, an Amazon.com Company

Contents

Foreword

He jests at scars that never felt a wound. – William Shakespeare[1]

You may find these pages hard to read sometimes. The information this book offers can be startling and shocking. Regardless of the reader's discomfort, this is an important book: it brings a vital message to us all about the dangers and traumas men and boys face from circumcision.

Add on to that the fact that the book is breaking one of Western culture's unwritten taboos: it talks openly about the emotional pain of men and boys. This taboo is rarely conscious and most people are simply unaware they even have it. I wouldn't have known about it but was confronted with it repeatedly in my psychotherapeutic work with men and boys for the last 30 years in helping them heal from trauma. It was blatantly apparent that no one wanted to hear the emotional pain of these men and boys. Most people would justify this by blaming the men as being cold and unfeeling. At first I wasn't sure what was happening, but over time it became clear. The emotional pain of men and boys is something that people will avoid like the plague. The men know this and act accordingly, taking care of their own emotional states by themselves.

It is this very taboo that helps us understand a bit more about circumcision. The taboo creates a situation where a man's emotional pain is avoided and a woman's emotional pain is a call to action. When we hear women in pain, we feel obligated to help in some way, to do something. When we hear about women facing the trauma of circumcision, we see it as an outrage and join forces to stop it in its tracks. But when we hear a man in pain, we turn it off. We don't hear it. "He can deal with it himself," we say to ourselves.

Our politicians are no different. They are very sensitive to women's pain and will draft legislation to try and be of help. That is how they get re-elected. But they do nothing for the men (and doing nothing for men rarely impacts their re-election). This, of course, is the situation we now face where female circumcision is outlawed in most western cultures in all its forms and is seen as a human rights violation. Meanwhile the circumcision of infant males is the most popular surgical procedure in America.

Since the emotional pain of men and boys is taboo and walled off, there is much less public concern for their pain than there is for that of girls and women. Almost every magazine or newspaper article you have seen on circumcision was probably about the circumcision of girls. If you look at the professional journals you will see a similar bias. There have been numerous journal articles about the traumatic psychological consequences of female circumcision, but I have yet to see one journal article about the psychological

---

[1] William Shakespeare, *Romeo And Juliet*, Act II Scene II.

7

consequences of the circumcision of males.[2] The articles that do appear are touting that male circumcision will prevent the disease of the day. Now it is HIV but the medical profession has sung this song before. They have assured us that male circumcision will prevent syphilis, epilepsy, spinal paralysis, bedwetting, eye problems, deafness, dumbness, tuberculosis, penile cancer, cervical cancer, and now HIV.

With the press framing women's circumcision as oppression and boys' circumcision as being healthy and life giving—and the medical profession doing much the same—it is little wonder that our general population will voice a very similar bias. Ask a random person on the street about female circumcision and they will tell you of the evil it takes to do such a thing, but ask them about boys and they will shrug their shoulders. They simply don't care, since they really don't know.

Reading this book will help you know. As you read this book you will be informed about the increasing awareness of the pain of men and boys as it relates to circumcision. We need more people with the courage to read this book and to then have an awareness of the pain of men and boys. We need this because without a sensitivity to a person's pain, there is no chance to offer compassion.

The world we live in is much less likely to render compassion for men and boys. This can change. You are changing it by reading this book. Thank you for your courage. The men and boys you love will thank you, too.

Thomas R. Golden, LCSW, author of *Swallowed by a Snake: The Gift of the Masculine Side of Healing* and *The Way Men Heal.*

13 March 2014

---

[2] There are a few articles on the psychological effects of circumcision on men but these are either not widely publicized or ignored. For example: T. A. Hammond, "Preliminary Poll of Men Circumcised in Infancy or Childhood," *British Journal of Urology International* 83, Suppl. 1 (1999): 85-92.

Acknowledgements

We are like dwarfs sitting on the shoulders of giants. We see more, and things that are more distant, than they did, not because our sight is superior or because we are taller than they, but because they raise us up, and by their great stature add to ours. – John of Salisbury (*Metalogicon*, 1159)

Those authors who have previously drawn attention to the harm of non-therapeutic circumcision of minors, including: Jim Bigelow, Lisa Bisque, Billy Ray Boyd, Robert Darby, Leonard Glick, Ronald Goldman, David Gollaher, Tim Hammond, Karen & John O'Hara, Patricia Robinett and Rosemary Romberg.

Psychotherapist Thomas Golden for suggesting this book.

The fifty courageous men from two foreskin restoration websites for telling their stories.[3]

Larry D. Wilson of San Jose, California, for his support and help in editing the text, particularly for his sensitive handling of men's stories.

Chris Ebbert, England, for 3D modeling and rendering of the illustrations.

Alison Tieman of Saskatchewan, Canada, for the cover art and design.

---

[3] foreskin-restoration.net and restoringforeskin.org

Dedication

As to immoral practice, it is hard to imagine anything more grotesque than the mutilation of infant genitalia. – Christopher Hitchens[4]

To the men and women who were deprived of normal sexual experience through the systematic genital reduction surgery carried out on them as children by the culture into which they were unfortunately born.

---

[4] Christopher Hitchens, *God Is Not Great; How Religion Poisons Everything* (Crows Nest: Allen & Unwin, 2007): 223.

Introduction

There is one category of men circumcised in infancy that most books, articles and studies about circumcision don't mention and whose existence most experts have not yet acknowledged: men who see themselves as victims of a mutilation but who are silenced by the humiliation, who would rather have their foreskins intact, but who cannot face the added humiliation of calling attention to the fact that part of their penis has been cut off.[5]

While society accepts that circumcision of girls produces harmful psychological effects, the medical profession and parents have been reluctant to acknowledge that the same applies to boys and men. Some men need emotional support to work through the pain of grief when they discover the truth about the physical and physiological harm of the non-therapeutic circumcision that was inflicted on them as non-consenting minors. The purpose of this book is to allow such men a safe place to speak out on this very personal topic. This book also encourages those who have ignored the pain to hear what these men are feeling.

The men range in age from eighteen to eighty-three and are from a wide range of educational and vocational backgrounds. Thirty-five of the men are from the United States, four from Canada, four from the United Kingdom and two from South Africa. Countries represented by one man each are New Zealand, Australia, Philippines, Iran and Iraq. With the exception of the Philippines, Iran and Iraq, where circumcision of minors has been culturally embedded for centuries, the other countries are primarily English speaking. Over a century ago in these countries, the medical profession started circumcising young boys to discourage masturbation.[6]

The word *Unspeakable* in the title of this book refers to the helpless infants and boys who during the circumcision procedure could not speak up in their own defense. *Unspeakable* also refers to the fact that the whole phenomenon of infant non-therapeutic circumcision is permeated with silence and the denial of harm, and when men do speak out about it, they are ridiculed. *Unspeakable* also refers to how hard it is for many men to even say out loud how hurt they are. Some circumcised men cannot even vocalize the word *circumcision.*

---

[5] J. Erickson, (1989) in Jim Bigelow, *The Joy of Uncircumcising, Exploring Circumcision: History, Myths, Psychology, Restoration, Sexual Pleasure and Human Rights* (Aptos: Hourglass Publishing, 2002): 52.

[6] Jews in English speaking countries have always been a very tiny proportion of the population.

When we want to hide from reality or deny something, we euphemize or soften the idea. Instead of saying *genital mutilation*, we say *circumcision*. We might find the term *uncircumcised penis* acceptable but would never use the term *uncircumcised vulva*. We find *mutilated penis* unacceptable only because Western society denies that male circumcision is in any way harmful because it is usually carried out in a clinical environment. To be able to confront this travesty, we must be able to describe it in accurate terms: It is an unnecessary destruction of a normal human body part.

Contrary to the belief of the majority within the medical profession, the foreskin is not "a flap of skin." It is, in fact, part of a very complex organ: the penis. It has layers, different parts and kinds of skin, and a range of functions. To this complexity must be added the fact that every circumcision is different: The result depends on the skill of the surgeon (often a beginning doctor), his/her experience, his/her attitude toward the operation, the type of instruments and methods used, etc. In addition, this is usually done when the penis is very small—after all, the weight of the infant will usually be about 6 pounds (3 kilograms). Thus, the impact of circumcision has many aspects, and the result may be very different for each man. There are, however, some common themes in the reactions of men to their circumcisions, many of which are revealed through their stories in this book.

Circumcision Coma

Most circumcised males never complain about having had their genitals surgically reduced. As in the case of female circumcision, such men accept what society tells them: it is healthier, culturally required, and more hygienic. Most circumcised men "are surprisingly ignorant of what has been done to them, and of course almost universally ignorant of what is normal."[7] In his story, Jeffrey suggests that such men are beguiled into a dream-like state not unlike that conjured by Morpheus.

Fortunately for themselves, their partners, their parents, those who circumcised them and society in general, most circumcised men happily spend their entire lives under Morpheus' spell and never realize that they have lost out sexually. This state of stupor is the *circumcision coma*.[8]

---

[7] Christopher Fletcher, "Penile Wounding: The Spectrum of Complications of Routine Male Circumcision as Seen in a Typical American Family Medical Practice," in *Genital Cutting: Protecting Children from Medical, Cultural, and Religious Infringements, edited by* George C. Denniston, et al., (Springer, New York/Heidelberg 2013): 85-99.

[8] David L. Gollaher, *Circumcision: A History of the World's Most Controversial Surgery* (New York: Basic Books, 2000): 180.

Introduction

Denial—The Shock Absorber

> Many [men] avoid any discussion of circumcision; others can discuss it only humorously. Some trivialize it, while others become angry when circumcision is challenged. To protect themselves from feelings of inferiority, many regard circumcision as "something done for them, not to them."[9]

Circumcised men typically deny they have suffered harm as a way of dealing with their shame. "Men have been perennially expected to do the providing and the protecting and our men are well aware of this expectation. This leads them to try and get the job done first and then emote on their own time and in their own space."[10] People blind from birth say they do not miss the ability to see. Similarly, most circumcised men say they do not miss having fully operational genitals. Perhaps the one exception is the circumcised adolescent boy, who soon learns the necessity of using a lubricant for masturbatory activities. It seems peculiar that males, who otherwise place significant value on their penis and its size, should reject the claim that they have a smaller penis and less sexual tissue. This is true denial—the *shock absorber*, since the anatomical evidence is indisputable.[11]

Men circumcised as babies "are cornered on this issue. They were circumcised without their consent and have no inherent knowledge of what being intact is like. … Men who have been circumcised have an extremely difficult dilemma. For them to acknowledge that the practice is unnecessary and harmful means that they must acknowledge a painful personal reality."[12] J. Rook says he remained in denial from age fourteen to seventeen. For some men, denial has persisted for decades before awakening from the circumcision coma. For most circumcised men the coma is lifelong, a state from which they never awaken.

Due to societal ignorance about foreskin functions, the loss of the foreskin

---

[9] T. A Hammond, "Preliminary Poll of Men Circumcised in Infancy or Childhood," *British Journal of Urology International* 83, Suppl. 1 (1999): 85-92.
[10] Thomas R. Golden, *The Way Men Heal* (Gaithersburg: G.H. Publishing, 2013) Kindle Edition. Golden's book is highly recommended for men undergoing circumcision grief and for those helping them.
[11] Thomas R. Golden, *Swallowed by a Snake: The Gift of the Masculine Side of Healing* (Gaithersburg: G.H. Publishing, 2000) Kindle Edition.
[12] Vincent Bach, "The Vulnerability of Men," http://www.stopcirc.com/vincent/vulnerability_of_men.html (accessed 7 April 2014).

may have no value or significance and so men deny *the meaning of the loss*.[13] This type of denial may also be expressed by saying "It's only a flap of skin," "I've never missed it," "It's more hygienic," "It's healthier," etc. Men block out any information that indicates that circumcision is equivalent to mutilation or process it using humor and accept the "values of the surrounding social environment."[14] Unsurprisingly, there is a strong parallel between male and female circumcision in maintaining this state of denial.

> ... the psychological effects are likely to be more subtle, buried beneath layers of denial, mixed with resignation and acceptance of social norms. ... they were forced to repress their feelings, banishing "consciousness," and even idealizing the custom, eventually justifying the procedure as harmless and necessary. ... [*They*] cannot recall their repressed anger and have never grieved about what happened to them. Consequently, they force the same ordeal on their children without wishing to acknowledge their action.[15]

Awakening—The Bad News

> I asked one day, posing it in a vague manner about things they might have done when I was born, and they mentioned I was circumcised. I pretended to act fine with it, and then just ... went up to my room to break down and cry for several hours in privacy.[16]

A man, or boy, can be awakened from the circumcision coma by comments from within or outside the family, interacting with intact males or, more commonly, today by information on the Internet. The awakening boy or man often experiences an unexpected and crushing recognition that he has a permanently and deliberately damaged penis.[17] Jeffrey writes that some men "are able to completely rip off the blinders that society imposes through lies of omission." He continues: "It really hit me as hard as a brick when I learned about all the parts removed." The *Global Survey of Circumcision Harm* reveals that anger (47%), shock (40%) and sorrow (35%) are common

---

[13] J. William Worden, *Grief Counseling & Grief Therapy* (New York: Springer, 1982), 11-12.

[14] Jim Bigelow, *The Joy of Uncircumcising!: Exploring Circumcision: History, Myths, Psychology, Restoration, Sexual Pleasure and Human Rights*, Electronic Edition, http://www.norm.org/ (2002): 111.

[15] T. A Hammond, "Preliminary Poll of Men Circumcised in Infancy or Childhood," *British Journal of Urology International* 83, Suppl. 1 (1999): 85-92.

[16] Someone Mundane at http://www.foreskinrestoration.net/forum/showthread.php?t=2961 (accessed 20 September 2009)

[17] T. A Hammond, "Preliminary Poll of Men Circumcised in Infancy or Childhood," *British Journal of Urology International* 83, Suppl. 1 (1999): 85-92.

emotional reactions.[18]

Shock, the state of numbed disbelief, protects the boy or man from being overwhelmed. This moment of awakening becomes encoded vividly and permanently in the memory. Jaime Banks "felt a flood of agony engulf" him. He "crawled into the walk-in closet" because he had nowhere else to hide. He sobbed and says he "felt his skin crawling all over [his] body, the vivid sensation of knives stabbing into [his] heart and abdomen. [He recalled] feeling as if malevolent, unseen entities were tearing at [his] flesh, consuming [him] alive."

Michael Gates remembers when he first heard about the "awful news" of the nerve loss caused by circumcision. He asks, "How awful is that feeling when your throat clenches and you need to act normal? When the seconds turn into minutes and the minutes into hours?" All he wanted to do was to go home and check the information, all the time hoping it was wrong. Greg at age fourteen "freaked the hell out and actually blacked out and ... remember[ed] suppressing the memory deep inside."

Disturbing New Information

From the Internet, circumcised boys and men can now easily find out that they have lost the most sensitive parts of their penis.[19] The very sensitive ridged band has been cut off and the frenulum damaged or removed entirely.[20] The most sensitive part of the penis to light touch is the tip of the foreskin.[21] Here the ridged band, containing thousands of nerve receptors called Meissner's corpuscles, functions to detect fine touch and movement, giving the man exquisitely pleasurable sensations. Lower densities of Meissner's corpuscles also occur in the glans corona.

---

[18] *Global Survey of Circumcision Harm,* http://www.circumcisionharm.org/ (accessed 13 December 2012)

[19] Gary Harryman, "The Lost List," http://www.norm.org/lost.html.

[20] J.R. Taylor, A.P. Lockwood and A.J. Taylor, "The Prepuce: Specialized Mucosa of the Penis and Its Loss to Circumcision," *British Journal of Urology* 77 (1996): 291-295; K. A. McGrath, "The Frenular Delta: a new Preputial Structure," in *Understanding Circumcision: A Multi-Disciplinary Approach to a Multi-Dimensional Problem,* edited by G.C. Denniston, F.M. Hodges, M.F. Milos (New York: Kluwer/Plenum, 2001): 199-206.

[21] J.R. Taylor, A.P. Lockwood and A.J. Taylor, (1996); Morris L. Sorrells et al. "Fine-touch pressure thresholds in the adult penis," *British Journal of Urology International* 99, 4 (2007): 864-869; K.A. McGrath, (2001).

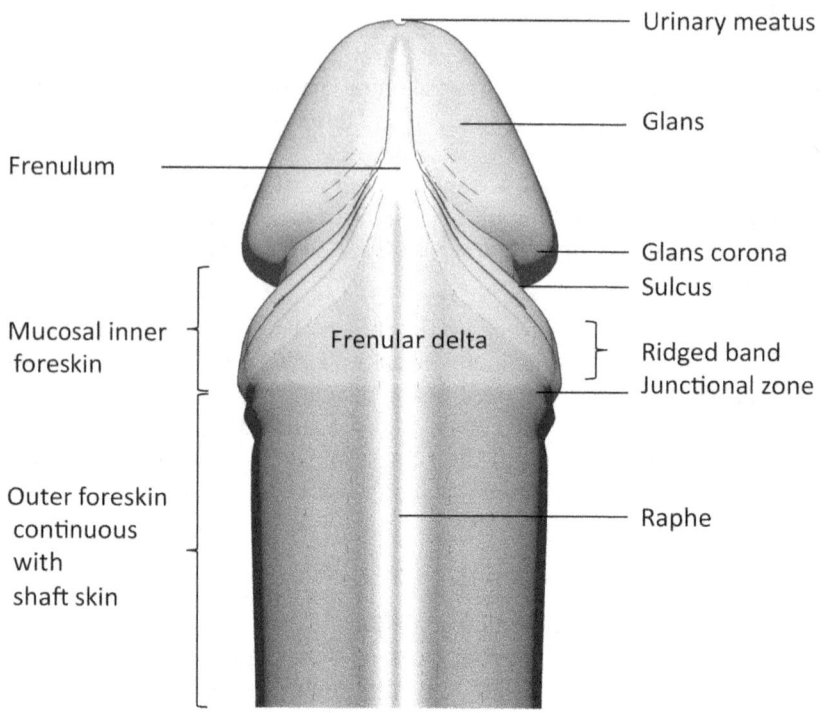

Fig 1: Underside of Penis with Foreskin Retracted

Predictably, because a 1.5 inch by 5 inch double layer of skin and muscle tissue has been cut off, circumcision results in a smaller penis. Normal men have a flaccid penis that is "5% longer, 4% bigger around, 15% larger in volume" than that of circumcised men.[22]

On awakening, scarring at the wound site suddenly becomes obvious. The Gomco Clamp[23] leaves a brown scar that encircles the penile shaft. There may be more obvious (hypertrophic) scarring where the scar stands out above the normal skin level. A skin tag (a non-functional mass of tissue) at

---

[22] Christopher Fletcher, "Penile Wounding: The Spectrum of Complications of Routine Male Circumcision as Seen in a Typical American Family Medical Practice," in *Genital Cutting: Protecting Children from Medical, Cultural, and Religious Infringements,* edited by George C. Denniston, et al. (Springer, New York/Heidelberg 2013): 85-99.

[23] The *Gomco Clamp* is a circumcision device developed by Hiram S. ('Inch') Yellen and Aaron A. Goldstein and used in the USA from 1935.

the injury site may then be recognized as a structural abnormality. Vance describes his private horror of living with a completely unnecessary and botched circumcision. Gary records how, because so much skin was removed during the circumcision he has had to live with a hairy penile shaft and penoscrotal webbing. Penoscrotal webbing is a common complication of circumcision in which, during erection, the skin of the scrotum is connected to the underside of the penis along a greater distance than is normal. This has destroyed Gary's confidence in relationships with women.

Men soon learn that the medical profession's assertion that circumcision makes no difference to sexual function is a deception, and that their sub-normal penile function may well be due to their infant circumcision. While not all male sexual dysfunction is due to circumcision damage, the surgeons who carry out the estimated 18,000 cases of circumcision corrective surgery in the United States each year must be aware of the physical damage of infant circumcision.[24] Even though this is only about 0.1 percent of the million plus circumcisions done to infant boys in the US each year, for every man affected, it means a subnormal sexual experience and reduced self-esteem. It is also a low estimate of serious penile damage, since many men with badly damaged penises will never seek corrective surgery.

Young Man from Canada reports that the urologist who removed his skin bridge said he had "done many, too many," indicating that skin bridge repair is not that uncommon among circumcised men. Parents may not be aware that their adult son has had corrective surgery to repair damage from their infant circumcision.

The recent American Academy of Pediatrics Task Force 2012 Report[25] provides an excellent sample of the old wives' tales, suppositions, disproven reasons for circumcision, superstition, bad science, and medical ignorance that helps to perpetuate this practice in America. Also, it should be pointed out, that the task force was very specific in its monetary goals: it recommended that all insurance and governmental programs should reimburse the doctors who perform this unnecessary operation.

Parents are easily caught up in this web of medical and cultural deceit. Chester from the Philippines, where circumcision is a custom forced on nearly all boys, tells how his parents said his foreskin should be cut off as it

---

[24] *Mens Health Magazine*, 2 May 2009, in Robert Darby, *The Sorcerer's Apprentice: Why Can't the United States Stop Circumcising Boys?*, Kindle Edition, SJF Publishing, 2013.
[25] American Academy of Pediatrics, "Male Circumcision," *Pediatrics* 130, 3 (2012): 756-785.

was "a medical danger" and with it he would "not be able to have sex at all," he would not be able to have children and that no girl would ever want to look at him naked. He was told that his "excess skin" was a divine mistake. Similarly in Iraq, groups of young boys are humiliated by having their genitals exposed and cut in public without pain relief, as described in Muslim Man's story. In his culture, speaking out against the genital mutilation of boys is forbidden; he must remain silent.

Nerve damage is caused by any surgical procedure and further trauma to the penile nerves may develop over time. Some circumcised men have a hypersensitive scar due to an over-supply of pain sensing nerve endings that develop at the injury site.[26] The constant stimulation of the exposed glans by clothing appears to diminish glans corona sensitivity. Hardly surprisingly, circumcised men often experience numbness and pain, since "... circumcision removes the most sensitive parts of the penis and decreases the fine-touch pressure sensitivity of the glans penis."[27] In his account, DPX1 describes how he felt minimal sensation when his partner carried out manual or oral sex on him.

Without the complete sensory input, ejaculation may be premature in circumcised young men or delayed in the middle aged. Orgasm may be simply an ejaculation rather than the full body orgasm experienced by the majority of men with whole genitals.[28] Without the foreskin's gliding property to reduce friction, circumcised males need to resort to using artificial lubricants for both masturbation and intercourse.[29] The high level of use of personal lubricants in Western circumcising countries confirms this.[30] Young American women, who are ignorant of the functions of the foreskin and have had little or no experience with intact men, often say they prefer cut

---

[26] M. Fitzgerald, "The birth of pain," *Medical Research Council News*, Summer (1998): 20-23.

[27] Morris L. Sorrells et al. "Fine-touch pressure thresholds in the adult penis," *British Journal of Urology International* 99, 4 (2007): 864-869.

[28] A.C. Kinsey, W.B. Pomeroy and C.E Martin, *Sexual Behavior in the Human Male* (Philadelphia: W.B. Saunders, 1948): 160-1.

[29] G.A. Bensley and G.J. Boyle, "Physical, sexual, and psychological effects of male infant circumcision: an exploratory survey," in *Understanding circumcision: a multi-disciplinary approach to a multi-dimensional problem,* edited by G.C. Denniston, F.M. Hodges and M.F. Milos (New York: Kluwer Academic/Plenum Publishers, 2001): 207–39.

[30] *Durex Global Sex Survey 2005*,http://www.durex.com/en-jp/sexualwellbeingsurvey/documents/gss2005result.pdf (accessed 6 October 2013).

partners. However, circumcised men may read research demonstrating that women who have experienced intercourse with both intact and circumcised men prefer intact. Circumcised men use longer and more vigorous strokes during intercourse to compensate for their missing penile sensory input.[31] Male circumcision is also correlated with "a range of frequent sexual difficulties in women, notably orgasm difficulties, pain during intercourse and a sense of incomplete sexual needs fulfillment."[32]

In summary, the awakened man soon learns that he will never be able to experience normal sexual function without the foreskin and its functions. The main functions are:

1. To provide pleasurable sensory input during sexual activities via the Meissner's corpuscles in the ridged band, the inner foreskin mucosa, and the frenulum.[33]

2. To protect the glans corona from abrasion, low air or water temperatures, and drying out, in order to preserve its limited sensitivity.

3. To protect the inner foreskin mucosa from abrasion and drying out, in order to maintain its sensitivity.

4. To provide enough skin for the erect penis to expand to its full erect volume without skin tears or bleeds.

5. To reduce the force needed to enter the vagina.[34]

6. To reduce friction between the penis shaft and the vaginal walls.[35]

7. To conserve vaginal fluids by acting as a barrier within the vagina.[36]

---

[31] K. O'Hara and J. O'Hara, "The effect of male circumcision on the sexual enjoyment of the female partner," *British Journal of Urology International* 83 Suppl. 1 (1999): 79–84.

[32] M. Frisch, M. Lindholm and M. Gronbaek, "Male circumcision and sexual function in men and women: a survey-based, cross-sectional study in Denmark," *International Journal of Epidemiology* (2011): 1-15. Accessed 18 June 2011. doi:10.1093/ije/dyr104.

[33] Morris L. Sorrells et al. "Fine-touch pressure thresholds in the adult penis," *British Journal of Urology International* 99, 4 (2007): 864-869.

[34] D. Taves, "The intromission Function of the Foreskin," *Medical Hypotheses* 59, 2 (2002): 180.

[35] R.L. Dickinson, Human Sex Anatomy: A Topographical Hand Atlas (Baltimore: Williams & Wilkins, 1949); S. Lakshmanan and S. Parkash, "Human prepuce: some aspects of structure and function," *Indian Journal Surgery* 44 (1980): 134-7.

[36] G.A. Bensley and G.J. Boyle, "Effects of male circumcision on female arousal and orgasm," *New Zealand Medical Journal* 116 (2003): 595-6.

Most men desire and expect their sexual experiences to be fulfilling and satisfying. Grief results because, due to the lack of a foreskin, this desire cannot be fully met, resulting in confusion, sadness, anger, fear, guilt, loneliness, or helplessness.

Anger

> I can't even begin to describe the feelings I had when I first learned ... rage, hatred, envy, disgust, sadness, feeling back-stabbed, feeling vengeful.[37]

> I felt completely overwhelmed by crushing despair and intense rage one day when I learned about it and after my suspicions were confirmed. I even exploded at my family.[38]

After awakening from the circumcision coma, 47% of men in the *Global Survey of Circumcision Harm* felt anger, and 27% reported "violent thoughts about and desire for retribution against [the] perpetrator."[39] J. Rook writes that on coming out of denial he entered a state of fury. Men feel they have been denied a completely fulfilling sexual experience. This parallels the reactions of victims of female circumcision, who feel deep anger, bitterness, and betrayal.[40] Anger comes from feeling helpless. This feeling intensifies because parents appear to have betrayed their son by neglecting to protect him. If the father is intact, the son can feel even greater betrayal. J. Rook's rage lasted for over a decade. Of course, it is better that anger is released safely or else resentment can simmer away for years as a "continuous smoldering bitterness."[41] Likely targets for circumcision hostility are parents, the medical profession, and religious leaders. CircVictim points out that babies are targeted because they are defenseless and that cutting an infant's genitals is a form of child abuse. The medical profession has very little appreciation of the intensity of hostility some circumcised men have towards circumcising doctors. Doctors "are evil greedy bastards hungry for money and power and don't have a millimeter of care in their whole body. Those

---

[37] IamJacksSmirkingRevenge at http://www.foreskin-restoration.net/forum/showthread.php?t=2585 (accessed 15 July 2009)

[38] Someone Mundane athttp://www.foreskin-restoration.net/forum/showthread.php?t=1361 (accessed 28 April 2011).

[39] http://www.circumcisionharm.org/ (accessed 13 December 2012)

[40] Nikki Denholm, *Female Genital Mutilation in New Zealand: Understanding and Responding – A Guide for Health and Child Protection Professionals*, (Auckland, The Refugee Health Education Programme, 2004): 70.

[41] R.M. Youngson, *Grief: Rebuilding Your Life After Bereavement* (Newton Abbot: David & Charles, 1989): 67; RPrizzle at http://www.foreskin-restoration.net/forum/showthread.php?t=2961 (accessed 20 September 2009).

who harm babies are pussy-like cowards and those who manipulate adults (as well as babies) have their name written on a bullet."[42] "I am angry because 28 years ago, I was only a defenseless newborn while some jackass doctor (or probably some bitch doctor) cut off my foreskin without any anesthesia."[43]

Some men develop images of extreme violence toward the circumciser and others involved in the cutting. "I am definitely angry at the doctor who cut me. I wish I could punch the hell out of him until he bleeds, then shove his head into a toilet full of shit, and crush his balls under my feet. I also hope he burns in hell."[44]

> I just want to hurt and/or kill the people involved with my circumcision, especially the one who actually performed it. ... I've thought about shooting them, choking them with metal wire, pushing them out of windows, beheading them, amputating the circumciser's penis so he's always horny but has no real way for release and so much more. ... I live in fear that one day the anger, rage and pain will consume me, but instead of plunging me into a deep depression it will drive me to the point of murder and suicide.[45]

Reactive Depression And Loneliness

> If we were talking about any other physical mishap or disease which had resulted in the amputation of a body part, the field of medicine and of psychology would not hesitate to recognize the validity of the problem and to help by whatever restorative and healing skills they had to offer.[46]

> ... the heart of it is the feeling that because my dick isn't as good as it could be, then I am not good enough and not worthy enough to be loved.[47]

One survey of awakened circumcised men revealed 42% of responders suffered from depressed periods or/and tearful breakdowns, and in another

---

[42] CircVictim at http://www.foreskin-restoration.net/forum/showthread.php?t=4852 (accessed 30 May 2010)

[43] Max Brown at http://www.myforeskin.org/content/milestones-and-anger-sep-1708 (accessed 26 December 2009).

[44] MaxBrown at http://www.myforeskin.org/content/milestones-and-anger-sep-1708 (accessed 14 March 2009).

[45] Aspie at http://www.foreskin-restoration.net/forum/showthread.php?t=5007 (accessed 7 June 2010).

[46] Jim Bigelow, *The Joy of Uncircumcising, Exploring Circumcision: History, Myths, Psychology, Restoration, Sexual Pleasure and Human Rights*, Electronic Edition, http://www.norm.org/ (2002): 116.

[47] UpwardsLemon at http://www.restoringforeskin.org/blog/2013/04/found-source-most-my-suffering-about-being-cut (accessed 21 April 2013).

survey 24% felt deep grief.[48] Grief consists of an individual's physical and mental responses to losing something valued, whether it be a person or a body part. Depression is a common response to such a loss. "One of the things that I still have to deal with is the depression the circumcision causes. Sometimes [the periods of depression] last hours, sometimes weeks and they hurt because contrary to popular belief depression doesn't equal deep sadness[. I]t equals a depression of the mind and body."[49] "I slept more often than normal. ... Nowadays though, I think all those extreme feelings have given way to a form of detached apathy as a coping mechanism. I find it difficult to *truly* care for anything anymore besides that, but I push myself to do so anyway. Doesn't always work, and it's kind of like a hollowed out feeling of caring, not really genuine."[50] Greg "went into a two-month psychotic breakdown" that destroyed him.

Not everyone with chronic depression becomes apathetic in order to deal with the pain. "I have been dealing with intense depression every day. Feeling of being inhuman, all the time, wearing me down. As I type this even, my body is trembling, eyes tearing up. Feel sick. This is pretty much a daily occurrence. I can't sustain a relationship because of it, even knowing the problem. And no matter what I do, I can't get over it. I've been on the strongest meds, legally and otherwise. I've tried therapy multiple times, all failing badly."[51] "I'm currently experiencing very real grief, about what was taken from me as an infant. ... I deal with all these new difficulties the only way I know how: One day at a time."[52]

A twenty-one year-old man explains:

> I get overwhelmed by feelings of sadness and anger and I sometimes break into tears. ... And these feelings haunt me in varying degrees throughout each and every day. I feel it when sex is mentioned in the media, I feel it when I look at myself in the shower or when I go to the bathroom. ... My emotional strength completely collapses, which is completely unacceptable

---

[48] http://www.restoringforeskin.org/poll/do-you-ever-have-any-tearful-breakdowns-andor-depressed-periods-because-your-circumcision (accessed 12 June 2012); http://www.circumcisionharm.org/ (accessed 13 December 2012).
[49] Aspie at http://www.foreskin-restoration.net/forum/showthread.php?t=5007 (accessed 7 June 2010).
[50] Someone Mundane at http://www.foreskin-restoration.net/forum/showthread.php?t=1361 (accessed 28 April 2011).
[51] Valentyne at http://www.restoringforeskin.org/forum/needing-get-stuff-my-chest (accessed 14 January 2011).
[52] Alfadog at http://www.foreskin-restoration.net/forum/showthread.php?t=7253 (accessed 18 April 2011).

at this point in my life. I have school and assignments to worry about, although I just don't know why I bother. I've already failed a couple of classes because of my depression and I'm on my way to a third.[53]

The awakened circumcised man grieves quietly and alone with little emotional support. "When he gets the message that people are uncomfortable talking about it, he is treated like it's not important or that he shouldn't question it, a man becomes aware of being cut off from society, and then a deeper circumcision of the soul sets in."[54] This echoes the plight of female circumcision victims who discover that because "there is often no acceptable means of expressing this pain, the women suffer in silence."[55]

> [Men] often think they are alone, and pretend contentment or indifference to save face, unaware that there are other circumcised men who have the same feelings and are pretending, too. Because they keep their thoughts and feelings to themselves, they are easy to be unaware of—and easy to ignore. That's one of the reasons infant circumcision can seem harmless—you rarely hear from or about the babies it eventually hurts the most.[56]

Usually men do not want to burden their parents or partners with their circumcision grief. "I can't talk to my mum about it because she is very sensitive and it will upset her, and I can't do that to her."[57] Thus, their concern about others close to them may contribute to furthering their isolation.

Some men, particularly the younger ones, have suicidal feelings. J. Rook recalls that he contemplated suicide. Brian Mathew Brandt, aged 28, committed suicide in 2012. Brandt "hated himself and his mother over a very aggressive circumcision conducted while he was an infant. This haunted him his whole life, as he explained to people that his was an aggressive circumcision gone wrong. He felt that he was mutilated and could never have sexual relations." He "tried to go through some courts, judges, and doctors

---

[53] Malparit23 at http://www.foreskin-restoration.net/forum/showthread.php?t=3477 (accessed 4 December 2009).

[54] T. Hammond, (1994) in David L. Gollaher, *Circumcision: A History of the World's Most Controversial Surgery* (New York: Basic Books, 2000): 180.

[55] Nikki Denholm, *Female Genital Mutilation in New Zealand: Understanding and Responding – A Guide for Health and Child Protection Professionals*, (Auckland, The Refugee Health Education Programme, 2004): 71.

[56] J. Erickson, (1989) in Jim Bigelow, *The Joy of Uncircumcising!: Exploring Circumcision: History, Myths, Psychology, Restoration, Sexual Pleasure and Human Rights* (Aptos: Hourglass Publishing, 1992): 52.

[57] Chrisalexander at http://www.foreskin-restoration.net/forum/showthread.php?t=5887 (accessed 4 October 2010).

only to have door after door shut on him—no one took him seriously. He wanted to get back at his mother for 'doing' this to him and thus saw suicide as the only way out."[58] Linda Massie writes of the attempted suicide of her twenty-year old son and how he "has never been able to form a sexual relationship, living a life of relative seclusion." This was the result of an unnecessary circumcision performed for phimosis when he was seven years old.[59] Phimosis is the inability of the foreskin to be retracted. It is rarely a pathological condition, although it is often misdiagnosed as such and treated with circumcision.

True Body Dysmorphia

In one survey 61% of responding men felt mutilated, 75% "felt less whole," and with "body dysmorphic disorder."[60] This longing for wholeness is a common experience and is not a passing feeling, but is life long. Such a reaction is similar to that experienced by amputees; they both experience anxiety, shock, grief, anger, depression, distrust, inhibitions, and feelings of inferiority.[61] Some men find the damaged appearance of their penis very difficult to accept.

> When I turned 22, I began foreskin restoration, but the appearance of the scar was too much. So, I took a heated metal flat to that area. I had a dark, wrinkly scar with skin tags, one the size of a pea. I hated what had been done to me. And I burned myself down there in hope to reduce the appearance. … So, in burning myself I reduced the appearance of the scar. I never completed that procedure. I reduced it by half. … The only way to make me feel less hurt is if I reduce the scar as much as I can and continue to restore my foreskin as much as I can, for as many years as it take[s]. … I want to be a man.[62]

Awareness of the shortcomings of the circumcised penis lowers self-esteem,

---

[58] http://www.nocirc.org/publish/NOCIRC_2012_nwsltr.pdf (accessed 10 July 2012). Quoted at http://foreskin-restoration.net/forum/showthread.php?p=84352 (accessed 9 February 2013).

[59] Massie, Linda, "Male Circumcision and the Potential for Unexplained Male Adolescent Suicide in Northern Ireland," in *Genital Cutting: Protecting Children from Medical, Cultural, and Religious Infringements,* edited by Denniston, George C.; Hodges, Frederick M.; Milos, Marilyn Fayre (Springer, New York/Heidelberg 2013): 101-6.

[60] http://www.circumcisionharm.org/ (accessed 13 December 2012).

[61] M. Bhojack, and S. Nathawat, (1988): 16-5 in Ronald Goldman, *Circumcision: The Hidden Trauma* (Boston: Vanguard Publications, 1997): 150.

[62] Sogious at http://www.foreskin-restoration.net/forum/showthread.php?t=4232 (accessed 14 March 2010).

so some men fear that they will be inadequate in performing sexual intercourse.[63] Some men avoid sexual intimacy as a result.

Awakened men can become obsessed with what is missing, since they are reminded every time they go to the toilet, take a shower, or engage in sexual activity. A survey at a foreskin restoration website revealed that 72% of respondents thought about their circumcision daily.[64]

While men circumcised as adults may be happier with their post-operative condition, not all are. Hatelife describes how he was supposed to have a biopsy, but the doctor removed his complete foreskin. As a result he started self-cutting and has been unable to sustain a sexual relationship.

Violation

> No pain would be greater than knowing what had been done to me, without anesthesia, against my will.[65]

One survey found 55% of men felt "violated or raped" and 37% felt shame.[66] This suggests a parallel with rape.[67] Both rape and the circumcision of minors involve restraint, and can be dehumanizing and terrifying. Rape survivors also experience guilt and shame, as well as anger and hostility towards the assailant. Some circumcised men have said they would rather have been raped, probably because rape does not remove a healthy body part.

> I think circumcision is indistinguishable from rape (a total violation of one's body and an affront to one's humanity), except that circumcision is perhaps worse in that it leaves both emotional and physical scars, and [physiological] crippling. And the whole "but you don't remember it, you were an infant" defense is as feeble and unpalatable as justifying date rape on the basis that a roofied woman won't remember what's done to her. It's mind-boggling to me how society can be so sympathetic toward the plight of raped women yet be so dismissive, and sometimes even ridiculing, toward the plight of circumcised men.[68]

---

[63] R. Goldman, *Circumcision: The Hidden Trauma* (Boston: Vanguard Publications, 1997): 142.

[64] Poll at http://www.restoringforeskin.org/poll/how-often-do-you-think-about-how-you-wish-you-had-not-been-circumcised-your-restoration- (accessed 7 July 2013).

[65] Sogious at http://www.foreskin-restoration.net/forum/showthread.php?t=4232 (accessed 14 March 2010).

[66] http://www.circumcisionharm.org/ (accessed 6 March 2012).

[67] T. A Hammond, "Preliminary Poll of Men Circumcised in Infancy or Childhood," *British Journal of Urology International* 83, Suppl. 1 (1999): 85-92.

Other Psychological Effects

> Since the event occurred at a very early preverbal level, it is most often experienced as a body or somatic memory rather than as a more familiar verbal memory. Various disturbing mental images and intense feelings often accompany the re-emergence of this body memory, including the feel of sharp metallic instruments cutting into one's flesh (anesthesia is normally not used in circumcision), the sense of being overpowered by big people, being alone and helpless, feelings of terror, and a sense of paralysis and immobilization. – John Rhinehart[69]

Some think that the body remembers the neonatal circumcision experience and Rick's story provides some evidence for this. It is also thought that infant circumcision can cause some men to experience dreams and nightmares. The connection between the two is not always made.

John Geisheker says:

> I have had a lifetime of vivid nightmares of being restrained and cut, and a terrible life-long fear of knives, to the extent that I cannot abide those magnetic knife holders some people use on their kitchen walls, which expose the blades all in a row. To be fair, the nightmares have faded as the years have gone by, and I cheerfully chop vegetables. At 60 years old, the worst nightmares only happen to me a manageable 3 or 4 times a year, though they are profoundly disturbing and take days to shake. ... The only sequelae, (clinical result), to use a physician's term, [from circumcision as a boy] is that I have the fastest 'vaso-vagal' reflex on the planet, able to faint dead-away at the mere combination of green walls, fluorescent light, the smell of isopropyl alcohol and the sight of lab coats. I have hit the floor upon the mere presentation of a tongue-depressor.[70]

Psychotherapists have been surprised when neonatal circumcision memories surface.

> When I first noticed this I was amazed and shocked ... I hadn't thought of the experience of circumcision as being anything but a routine medical procedure. The men who re-lived things were usually just as startled. They

---

[68] IamJacksSmirkingRevenge at http://www.foreskin-restoration.net/forum/showthread.php?t=2585 (accessed 8 July 2009). *Roofied* describes a person who has suffered a sexual assault facilitated by use of drug-induced amnesia.

[69] J. Rhinehart, "Neonatal circumcision reconsidered," *Transactional Analysis Journal* 29, 3 (1999): 215-21.

[70] John Geisheker at http://www.genitalintegrity.net/blouch/2006/07/ (accessed 2 January 2008, no longer available).

were usually expecting other issues to surface and were surprised to see circumcision as one of them. We were both shocked at the intensity of the related pain. I started looking into the medical aspects and was completely blown away to find that doctors didn't use any anesthetic ... the assumption being that babies don't feel pain. ... I checked with other therapists doing this sort of work and folks who had written about this and found that it was not an uncommon experience.[71]

Among his patients John Rhinehart found "serious and sometimes disabling lifelong consequences" that appear to have resulted from neonatal circumcision. This is a type of Delayed Post Traumatic Stress Disorder (PTSD), characteristic of people abused as children.[72] PTSD seriously interferes with a person's life and lasts longer than a month.[73] For men the commonest traumatic events that cause PTSD are rape, combat experiences, or neglect or physical abuse in childhood.[74] The event must be overwhelming, threatening to one's body, unexpected, and cause "fear, helplessness, or horror in the person involved."[75] Circumcision of babies and boys clearly fits these criteria, as Muslim Man's experience demonstrates. PTSD symptoms include nightmares, emotional detachment, numbing of feelings, insomnia, avoidance of reminders, extreme distress when exposed to triggers, loss of appetite, irritability, hyper-vigilance, memory loss, startle response, depression, and anxiety.

Specific cues or triggers remind the man of the circumcision trauma, resulting in a flight or fight response. Examples of circumcision triggers are: babies; a baby crying; hospital sights, smells and sounds; the physical sensations associated with foreskin restoration; sexual intercourse; the sight of their own circumcised penis while urinating or bathing; men with intact genitals; birthdays, etc. For example Tormod "cringed and broke into a sweat" whenever he heard the word "circumcision." Bill Sloan recalls that any word with the prefix "circ" brings back "all the horror" of circumcision to him, while the prefix causes J. Rook to "nearly boil over with rage." Normally, PTSD victims avoid reminders of the original trauma and if exposed to the stimulus can have a strong physiological reaction. "A couple of years ago I watched one of those [circumcision] videos. It was a mistake. I

---

[71] http://www.menweb.org/circtom.htm (accessed 12 December 2007).

[72] J. Rhinehart, "Neonatal circumcision reconsidered," *Transactional Analysis Journal* 29, 3 (1999): 215-21. Rhinehart gives four examples from his clients.

[73] Mark Goulston, *Post Traumatic Stress Disorder for Dummies*, (New Jersey, Wiley, 2008): 27-29.

[74] ibid., 17.

[75] ibid., 22.

sicked up on the floor beside the computer. Now, I have seen some horrible bloody sights in Belfast in the last 30 years. But we tried to help and comfort the victims. No sign of comfort in these images of circumcision torture."[76]

It is now known that circumcised men experience more difficulty identifying and describing feelings (alexithymia) than intact men.[77] Perhaps this partially explains why circumcised men are so comfortable taking on the role of circumcisers or having their sons circumcised. Alexithymia may make it more difficult for a man to break out of the circumcision coma and to work through the grief process.

Confronting Parents

Part of the healing process for circumcised men is for their parents to acknowledge that circumcision has caused physical and mental distress. Unless parents have been physically and verbally abusive, most circumcised men exclude them from blame, since they were trying to do their best and were ignorant of the consequences of their actions. In fact, many men want to avoid hurting their parents, despite the emotional pain caused by the parents' action. Because the physical and mental damages are irreversible, a sincere apology and ongoing support through the grief are the best that parents can offer.

Conversations with parents can be lengthy and emotionally tense for both sides, and the result is not predictable. Canaanite had a lengthy conversation via Skype with his parents. While it was an emotional interaction, all participants came out of the encounter with a more positive relationship. In comparison, Joseph from Oregon just wanted his parents to apologize, but they would not. Bigelow believes honesty between both parents and the son "might well heal breaches in the family structure that many parents do not even know exist."[78] He reports that most men "have never discussed their circumcision or their feelings about it with their parents."[79] As part of their healing process most men prefer an active path and so may be uncomfortable

---

[76] Tormod - IRL at http://www.foreskin-restoration.net/forum/showthread.php? t=2621 (accessed 26 July 2009).

[77] Dan Bollinger and Robert S. Van Howe, "Alexithymia and Circumcision Trauma: A Preliminary Investigation," *International Journal of Men's Health* 10, 2 (2011): 184-195.

[78] R. Goldman, *Circumcision: The Hidden Trauma* (Boston: Vanguard Publications, 1997): 199-200.

[79] Jim Bigelow, *The Joy of Uncircumcising, Exploring Circumcision: History, Myths, Psychology, Restoration, Sexual Pleasure and Human Rights* (Aptos: Hourglass Publishing, 1992): 106-7.

using the "cry and discuss" strategy with anyone, let alone parents. Also, confronting parents about a part of their genitals is not easy for men, especially when the parents' reaction is more likely to be negative and trivializing rather than compassionate. In a similar way to their sons, parents also have to undergo a healing process in which they must process the consequences of their circumcision decision. In this way, the psychological effects of circumcision affect the emotional climate of the whole family.

As in the case of Alfadog, sons are more likely to approach their mothers (40%) than their fathers (25%), and mothers are more likely to be more apologetic and less dismissive than fathers.[80] From the parents' viewpoint such a revelation from the son comes unexpectedly, although the son may have been planning the conversation for months or even years. Commonly on foreskin restoration websites men discuss the pros and cons of confronting their parents with the "why?" question. Some parents think it peculiar that a son would even question their circumcision decision. The complete lack of compassion and the expression of anger from parents greatly puzzles grieving men, leaving them feeling even more alone and alienated. Jeffrey tells how he "felt abandoned by the only people that I should always feel I could turn to. My mother, life herself, refused to cradle and comfort me like the baby she always considers me."

Parental rejection is particularly difficult for teenagers to cope with. A fourteen-year old boy found that "instead of showing compassion, my parents ended up being angry at me for even questioning them, and my dad acted like I had insulted him. They still don't understand, and I haven't talked about it with them since then. ... It's rough. It hurts like hell, and the hurt isn't going to go away quickly.'[81]

Sometimes the interaction results in a complete standoff. The parents refuse to acknowledge that their actions have caused harm and the son feels too insecure emotionally to continue raising the issue because he will be ridiculed or put down. A rift develops and this may endure for years. Since telling his parents how he felt about being circumcised, TopHat says he has had a non-existent relationship with them.

In Mikey's father's reply, we read that his father did what he thought was best for his son, motivated by a strong fear of sexually transmitted infections. This probably reflects the misinformation that the medical profession was spreading at the time. Mikey is grateful for his father's honest reply, but

---

[80] http://www.circumcisionharm.org/ (accessed 6 March 2012).
[81] Moniker at http://www.foreskin-restoration.net/forum/showthread.php?t=3312&page=2.

obviously wants to educate his father further. Mothers, like their circumcised husband and sons, also become victims. They are vulnerable to an assertive circumcised husband or intrusive relations and, particularly in America, bullying medical professionals. Of course, the circumcised husband pushes the circumcision of his son to avoid confronting his own penile inadequacy, but the mother is ignorant of this and believes the husband knows best about penile matters. A young father is unlikely to be aware of the sensitivity loss he will experience as he approaches middle age and, after all, he is able to perform adequately during his early adult life when he is required to produce offspring.

Unfortunately, it is the mother who bears the major burden of guilt when she discovers that the procedure is both damaging and unnecessary and that she has not protected her baby from harm. Alfadog discovered his mother crying as a result of an earlier conversation he had with her. If the circumcision is "botched," parents are thrown into confusion because their flawless baby has been damaged for unconvincing reasons. Mothers often express feelings of inadequacy that they failed to protect their son. "My son is now 35 years old and I really still regret it. A few years ago he asked me why I had him circumcised at birth, why I bothered to do that, why I didn't just leave it alone? I had no answers. I told him that I had regretted it many times and I was sorry even now. He harbors no bad feelings toward me, but I know he wishes he were intact."[82]

Male Healing

> It has been said, "time heals all wounds." I do not agree. The wounds remain. In time, the mind, protecting its sanity, covers them with scar tissue and the pain lessens. But it is never gone. – Rose Kennedy[83]

> You can never fully get rid of it but you learn to live with it.[84]

It is commonly said that men never complain or show emotions about having been circumcised. This is to be expected, because, as Kohiro notes, "as men we are taught to not express our emotions." A man is supposed to provide and protect, not be needy or dependent. Males are supposed to be at the top of an invisible dominance hierarchy, along with the physically strong male sports heroes. Any man who complains is likely to be ridiculed.

---

[82] Gitti at http://www.mothering.com/discussions/showthread.php?t=112410 (accessed 14 August 2010) This website contains many testimonies from mothers who regret their circumcision decision.

[83] http://www.quotationspage.com/quote/39132.html (accessed 22 November 2009).

[84] rmcj on a discontinued website (accessed 2 February 2010).

Compared to women, men have different hormonal and brain chemistry systems, and men must work through grief using their unique male faculties. Golden says male grieving is typically silent and usually goes unrecognized. Most men feel more comfortable working through grief using *action* rather than crying and talking. *Creative action* might involve creating artworks, writing poems as Kohiro and Jaime Banks have done, making or improving foreskin restoration devices or writing replies to circumcision blogs.[85] In his account, Greg B explains how he became a moderator on several circumcision forums after discovering the harm of circumcision.

Practical action[86] might involve foreskin restoration, performing music, confronting parents or the circumciser, or making a pilgrimage to the hospital. Some men join the growing number of *intactivists* and actively promote the concept that both male and female minors have a right to intact genitals. Ron tells how he used his skills to make his own restoring device and gradually developed a full time business that has sold thousands of devices to restoring men. Practical action is more difficult in the case of a personal body part than for a dead person. With the latter we can hold funerals or celebrations, set up gravestones, and discuss or write about the person's achievements. Such actions are not so appropriate in the case of circumcision grief, although there are rare exceptions.

> I told my girlfriend about all this stuff two days ago, and all the emotion came out. I actually cried when I told her that I just wanted to feel whole and unashamed of my penis. She gently held me in her arms and told me that she was proud of me, loved me no matter what my penis looks like, and would do anything to help me out. Then her and some of our friends placed their hands on me and prayed to Jesus for the recovery of my foreskin and sensitivity (this was definitely the oddest prayer circle I've been in but, hey, you can't find friends more supportive than this). I don't have any anger towards my parents or anything. I just want what is mine back.[87]

Thinking action might involve any process that exposes the man's feelings, and could involve keeping a journal, writing a letter to parents or the doctor, reading books on grief or even meditation. Alternatively there is *inaction*, involving self-reflection to process thoughts when the man is quiet and alone.[88]

---

[85] Thomas R. Golden, *The Way Men Heal* (Gaithersburg: G.H. Publishing, 2013) Kindle Edition.

[86] ibid.

[87] http://www.newforeskin.biz/members/framesetMain.htm (accessed 30 June 2007)

Grief may be intense and healing may be protracted for a circumcised man because he naturally has a strong attachment to his penis and his lost foreskin, he was unprepared for the revelation that circumcision was done and/or the extent of the subsequent damage, he perceives circumcision as completely unnatural, he regards his penis as constituting a very significant part of his sexual identity, and he depends on a complete penis to experience optimal sexual pleasure.[89] There is also the desensitized glans and the ugly scarring, both constant reminders of the missing part. For some men acceptance of the injury done to them by an unsympathetic medical profession through the betrayal of ill-advised parents may hardly seem possible. However, as J. Rook found, for some men it is possible to pass through the grief and progress along a "path to forgiveness and empathy."

There is a group of circumcised men who, before they awakened, allowed their sons to be cut as well and have to face up to what they did to their sons. Restore1 tells why his first son was cut, but his younger one was not. Because of his open and sensitive relationship, he was able to discuss the matter with both his sons and this helped assuage his guilt. Awakened fathers in this group carry a lifelong burden of guilt.

Helping Men Grieve

> Most men come from a background of never having had someone show an interest in their emotional pain. – Thomas Golden

Goldman says: "Generally, the importance of the support of women cannot be overestimated. Female understanding and compassion are vital to men as they feel increasingly sensitive and vulnerable to feelings about circumcision. The rewards for this support can be considerable for both men and women."[90] An example of partner support is exemplified by the following: "I have been married to the Oregon Intactivist for fourteen years and can tell you being circumcised has haunted him more than people will ever know. If your husband says he doesn't like being circumcised, it is not a joke. Males deserve to be left intact the way they're born and to enjoy sex as God intended."[91]

---

[88] Thomas R. Golden, *The Way Men Heal* (Gaithersburg: G.H. Publishing, 2013) Kindle Edition.

[89] Based on concepts in Thomas R. Golden, *Swallowed by a Snake: The Gift of the Masculine Side of Healing* (Gaithersburg: G.H. Publishing, 2000) Kindle Edition.

[90] R. Goldman, *Circumcision: The Hidden Trauma* (Boston: Vanguard Publications, 1997): 200.

To support a typical man in the circumcision grief process:[92]

1. Help him to maintain his independence.
2. Let him know he is respected and admired. His self-esteem may be low because he is incomplete and he may feel shame or sexual inadequacy because his penis is incomplete.
3. Support him in the activity he chooses to process grief. For example: foreskin restoration.
4. Honor his loss without judgment or making justifications for what was done to him.
5. Talk about his actions and not his feelings.
6. Expect black moods, irritability and anger. Having been circumcised against one's will is a gross invasion of bodily integrity that is equivalent to rape.

Active Grieving: Foreskin Restoration

Recognizing that deep conflicts and anxieties have existed for a reason and are a proper response to the early trauma can also contribute to healing. Surviving early trauma is a triumph for the human spirit. – Ronald Goldman[93]

As part of an active grieving process some men engage in non-surgical foreskin restoration. This may not be recognized as part of the healing process and sometimes men even hide it from their partners. Foreskin restoration allows men to grow more skin and improve appearance, function and pleasure. Several methods are used to apply gentle tension to the foreskin to stimulate skin growth through cell division.

Manual: Using the hands to apply tension is cheap and it allows the uneven skin remnants to be corrected. Manual restoration is often the first method, but can be used to achieve a complete restoration.

Cross Taping: The foreskin remnant is stretched up over the glans and held in place with strips of surgical tape to apply tension. This method is usually used in the early stages.

---

[91] http://oregonintactivist.com/circumcision-stories/oregon-intactivist/ (accessed 25 September 2013) Used with permission.
[92] Based on Thomas R. Golden, *The Way Men Heal* (Gaithersburg: G.H. Publishing, 2013) Kindle Edition.
[93] R. Goldman, *Circumcision: The Hidden Trauma* (Boston: Vanguard Publications, 1997), 199.

Advanced Taping: The tape is applied and various means are employed to apply tension. Examples include using elastic straps, inserting foam or silicon cylinders inside the growing skin tube, taping the skin to tubes and then pulling on the tube or stuffing cotton into the tube.

Devices: If there is sufficient remnant foreskin, a device (either homemade or commercial) can be used to apply tension. Some devices apply tension using a weight or strap, while others are designed to push against the glans. Both homemade and commercial variations are used. Soon designs will be available for 3D printers.

Inflation: Modeled on the methods used by plastic surgeons to grow skin, tension is applied to the skin tube using air or water-filled balloons. Both homemade and commercial variations are used.[94]

Foreskin restoration does not remove scarring or restore the sensitivity of the missing ridged band and frenulum (often also cruelly removed by American doctors) that have evolved to be the sites of much sensory input and pleasure. However, foreskin restoration can result in greater sensitivity of the glans corona, frenulum (if present) and the inner mucosa, increased mobility and pleasure of the new mucosa moving over the corona, a more normal appearance, a more natural covering of the glans, and an almost normal gliding mechanism that reduces friction during intercourse.[95] After restoring, some men, like Greg B, report having *full body orgasms* for the first time in their lives, rather than just experiencing ejaculations. "Now, I have orgasms. They are much more intense and it usually takes me several minutes to recover and catch my breath. In other words, I used to ejaculate; now I have orgasms."[96] J. Rook observes that "restoring completes healing." Some men also report a positive result for their partners. Swampthing, for example, records how three years after starting restoration his wife no longer experiences any pain from intercourse.

---

[94] From notes supplied by Gregory Breese.
[95] Jim Bigelow, *The Joy of Uncircumcising!: Exploring Circumcision: History, Myths, Psychology, Restoration, Sexual Pleasure and Human Rights* (Aptos: Hourglass Publishing, 1992), 138.
[96] Tally at http://www.foreskin-restoration.net/forum/showthread.php?t=2029 (accessed 7 April 2009).

Confronting the Unspeakable

> *The Victim's Narrative*: The story begins long before the harmful act, which was just the latest incident in a long history of maltreatment. The perpetrator's actions were incoherent, senseless, incomprehensible. Either that or he was an abnormal sadist, motivated only by a desire to see me suffer, though I was completely innocent. The harm he did was grievous and irreparable, with effects that will last forever. None of us will ever forget it. – Steven Pinker[97]

The contributors to this book have not only confronted what has been done to their sexuality, but have been willing to share it with us. We thank them for their willingness to tell us about some very personal experiences and feelings. We especially thank them for helping to try to protect others from the damage that they have received through their unspeakable mutilations.

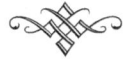

---

[97] Steven Pinker, *The Better Angels of our Nature: the Decline of Violence in History and its Causes* (London: Penguin, 2011), 489.

When Cut Men Speak Out

When cut men speak out
They express their sense of loss.
Their message is lost.

When cut men speak out
They express their betrayal.
No one wants to hear.

When cut men speak out
They express their resentment.
Just get over it.

When cut men speak out
They express their enragement.
People laugh at them.

So cut men don't speak
Their pain is hidden away.
Cutting continues.

Thomas
38 years
Florida, USA
10 April 2014

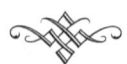

A Few Dollars. A Lifetime Scar.

There are no valid medical indications for circumcision in the neonatal period.[98]

I was born on 28 September 1975 in Concord, Massachusetts. My mother was seventeen at the time, and my father was a nineteen-year-old, enlisted in the US Air Force. I'm told that it was a beautiful autumn day, and all went well.

After I was delivered by the obstetrician, I was examined by a pediatrician. I'm told that he was about fifty years old and a snappy dresser. This is all I know about this man, all I will ever know about this man as the records are not kept longer than twenty years. There was nothing at all the matter with me: I was a healthy baby boy.

However, the pediatrician, for reasons that I will never know, found my penis objectionable. This was an issue of great concern to him. I had a pretty, perfect penis, with a prepuce, and he was determined to deprive me of it. My parents, on the other hand, were not worried about it. They didn't feel there was a reason to do anything to my penis. My mother told the pediatrician, "No." He became very annoyed with her.

He came back the next day to press the issue; he insisted that I'd want to be like my father. (Years later when I argued with my wife, she stung me by saying, "You're being just like your father.") My mother relented because this high status, well-dressed doctor was determined, and she would stand in his way no longer. On 30 September 1975, a Tuesday, I was strapped into a Circumstraint, positioned hips elevated, with my penis perfectly presented to the pediatrician. I could not understand, consent, refuse or escape. No analgesia would have been used. The intense pain that I was to endure would have a lasting impact on my neurological development. Unperturbed by my pain, the pediatrician proceeded.

There is no absolute medical indication for routine circumcision of the newborn.[99]

What were this man's motivations? Why was it so important to him what my penis looked like? Why did he think that the most intimate part of my body,

---

[98]American Academy of Pediatrics Committee on Fetus and Newborn. *Standards and Recommendation for Hospital Care of Newborn Infants*. 5th ed. (Evanston: American Academy of Pediatrics, 1971), 110.
[99] H.C. Thompson, L.R. King, E. Knox, et al. "Report of the ad hoc task force on circumcision," *Pediatrics* 56, 4 (1975): 610-1.

my "private parts," my penis, was his prerogative? I'll never know what he wanted from me. But whatever it was, he took it.

He got what he wanted. He had his way with me. He carved his paycheck into my penis. He carved his religion into my penis. He carved his tribal marking into my penis. He carved his custom into my penis. He carved his grotesque esthetic preferences into my penis. He carved his obscene signature into my penis. He carved his sadistic sexual fetish into my penis.

My mother thinks that the pediatricians' predilection for pruning the prepuce from penises was primarily pecuniary. I look at the scar on my penis, and wonder, "What is this?" A night out on the town—flushed down a toilet. A pair of wing-tip shoes—at the bottom of a landfill since 1978. A golf club—sold at a yard sale in 1983. Whatever enjoyment he had was fleeting; it's long gone. But 38 years later, the scar is still on my penis, and will be until the day I die—and for what?

In the film *Robin Hood, Men in Tights*, Mel Brooks plays a mohel[100] who attempts to sell circumcisions to a group of twenty-somethings. His pitch, "The ladies love it, the men all want it." Then he explains the procedure, and the men want none of it. He concludes, "I gotta work a much younger crowd."

While I will never really know the motivations of my assailant, I'm chillingly aware of why it had to be done to me in infancy. He would never see me again, he would never need to know what I thought of his work, he would never have to face me, he would never need to answer for what he has done. This is the reason, for there is no valid medical reason that this is the best time.

There are lots of medical reasons that this is a bad time. My prepuce was fused to my glans, and he tore them apart. Anesthetic is dangerous; he would have used none. My penis grew much larger and he could not know what the final result would be. He had to do it to me in infancy to exercise power over me, to deny me the opportunity to refuse, to deny me any memory of the pretty perfect penis with prepuce that I was born with, to hide the assault from me—as though I were just born that way. Most of all because it's so easy to say yes—when it's not your penis.

---

[100] A *mohel* is a Jewish ritual circumciser.

If the benefits of circumcision were compelling, competent well-informed men would choose it for themselves, but very few normal men do. Only 1 in 3000 genitally intact American men will request circumcision as an adult for non-medical reasons. The rates are even lower in Europe.[101]

They could hide the memory, but the scar will always be on my penis, and they could not hide what they did to me forever. When I was six years old, my bother and I were peeing into a toilet with my friend Lucas. I noticed that there was something different about Lucas's penis, it had skin all the way down and tapered at the tip. His urine sprayed out, rather than coming out in a defined stream. I didn't know why, or what to think. My younger bother noticed too. But he took the next step—he asked about it.

I'll never forget that day. I was standing in the small backyard of our condo in San Diego, when he opened the glass door and announced, cryptically, that "they" cut off something that "could cause infections." I had no idea what he was talking about. I remained oblivious, but an impression had been made.

Circumcision ablates the most sensitive parts of the penis.[102]

In 1993 I was a junior in high school. Howard Stern, the shock jock, was on the airwaves, and, boy, was I in for a shock—even though I never listened to his show. My friend Nathan did. One night, Nathan said to me, "That's the most sensitive part."

One angst filled sentence. I still didn't really know what had been cut off. That one angst filled sentence would ring in my ears for years to come. I was upset. He was upset. I was upset, simple as that. Why was I upset? I didn't know anything about the prepuce, or why it was important, or really even what it meant to be "the most sensitive part."

What did I know? I knew that it was my penis. I knew that I wasn't given a choice.

I knew that I was upset. I knew that my friend thought it had value. I knew that it had value because it was mine. I knew that I wanted it back.

---

[101] J.S. Svoboda, "Circumcision of Infants as a Human Rights Violation," *Journal of Medical Ethics* 39, 7 (2013): 469-474.
[102] Morris L. Sorrells et al. "Fine-touch pressure thresholds in the adult penis," *British Journal of Urology International* 99, 4 (2007): 864-869.

I knew that what little I knew was enough to know that it was wrong. Thus began a decades long journey to undo what my assailant did in minutes.

Thomas
38 years
Florida, USA
5 December 2013

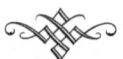

A Reprieve From Shame: A Journey Through Time

I was conceived shortly before WWII in a small house in a small town located on a dry, dusty, Dakota plain.

Seven months later, on the last legs of their round-the-world trip, authors Christopher Isherwood and W. H. Auden rolled through the little town, the hot railway tracks on which their railway car moved lying within a block of where I lay quietly in my mother's womb. Isherwood characterized their foray through the State as a "dismaying contrast" to their pleasant journey through the Canadian Rockies. "The hot shabby prairie was blowing itself away in clouds of dust," he quipped. Would that I might have been able to reach out and touch their liberating presence. Alas, that close encounter with Isherwood would not be repeated for another thirty-five years.[103]

My birth occurred fifteen miles away, on a hot August morning, in another not-quite-so-small town, in a little hospital run by a Catholic Order of Nuns. I was left intact at birth, circumcision being a procedure virtually unknown to the attending physician, who was an old-time Norwegian doctor.

Considering that people were being slaughtered throughout the world, my childhood was relatively quiet and uneventful. However, when I was about twelve to thirteen years old a friend and I were walking together to our respective homes at lunchtime. Just prior to my turning off, my friend stopped for a minute and asked a question that would change my life forever, a question that brought me up short. He asked me if I had been circumcised, or if I had a foreskin.

Now this was a subject that was completely foreign to me—a subject that had never before entered my consciousness. Though by that time I had experienced several innocent childhood sexual encounters, sexual matters were never discussed in our home. I was completely unconscious of sex. We were brought up to be shame-based, and it was impossible to ask questions in our home.

By that time I had heard the term "circumcision," but I had no first-hand knowledge of what it meant. Therefore, I had to stop and think of what to say, what to tell my friend. After hesitating an embarrassing moment or two, I managed to mumble, "Yes, I'm intact," with my fingers crossed, because I really wasn't sure.

---

[103] The Isherwood/Auden journey is mentioned in Christopher Isherwood, *Christopher and His Kind: 1929-1939* (New York, Farrar, Straus Grioux, 1976), 313.

"I am, too," Friend exclaimed, a big smile on his face. "But I can skin mine back," he continued, proudly.

My mind immediately registered everything. He *knew*! I could only guess that a cousin had told him that I couldn't retract. However, that possibility was an entirely new concept for me—something foreign, something unanticipated, something completely unknown. So, I told myself, I had a foreskin, but it was supposed to retract. It was a shock: startling. Friend went on and on about how much he enjoyed "playing" with his foreskin. Had I not been so shame-based, perhaps I would have inquired about it, asked to compare, instituted a show-and-tell or something. However, this new knowledge devastated me—made me feel less than whole: embarrassingly "different."

Humiliated, I peeled off and walked home. Going behind our garage, I pulled out my penis and for the first time closely examined the mysterious foreskin … and, yes, inside its tiny quarter inch opening I could see a small portion of a shiny surface ... what I later learned was my glans penis. Inside I could see my piss-slit ... the meatus ... and noticed that the two openings did not line-up. Finally, I discovered why it was difficult to urinate without spraying all over the place ... why it was so much more convenient to urinate from a seated position. I managed to get an erection, and saw clearly that that only made the situation worse, the shaft skin pulled so tight that my penis was severely constrained.

So, what to do?

It would have been impossibly embarrassing to talk to my parents. I thought of going alone to see our doctor, now the son of the physician who had attended my birth. That in itself would have been embarrassing. I was intelligent enough to know that he would probably advise circumcision. Having heard my friend speak enthusiastically about the pleasures he felt while moving his foreskin, I couldn't see how circumcision would benefit me. I was in a quandary of wanting to have a functional foreskin, but unable to see how that might be achieved.

It was then I decided to wait: to wait until I was away from home to independently consult a doctor, who surely would know what needed to be done. Why I would think that is a puzzle, considering that prior to my discovery I had been examined by dozens of doctors, some of them eminent physicians at the Mayo Clinic, about a different physical condition. Never had a single doctor looked at or examined my penis up-close, and so they were just as ignorant as me. Was it shame that prevented them from looking? Fear? Ignorance?

After leaving home, that's exactly what I did—went from doctor to doctor, seeking a solution to the problem of my very tight foreskin and its tiny opening. Every time a physician examined my penis they, without exception, immediately advised circumcision. They could advise no other solution. By that time my foreskin problem was having unforeseen consequences in my social/sexual life, too. Whenever I got close to another person, the embarrassment and shame of my situation paralyzed me.

Eventually my despair became so acute that I very reluctantly acquiesced to the latest physician who recommended circumcision. He made an appointment, and I submitted myself to the knife. It was the worst decision of my life, one I regret every single day.

Evidently the dirty deed was done by a doctor-in-training, as there were two of them, one giving directions, the other apparently cutting, though I could see nothing, a curtain having placed in front of my face. The result was and is not very pretty: large skin tags attached to the corona, concealing much of the sulcus, a blob-like remnant of my frenulum, and even now, decades later, periodic bleeding from the scars. Immediately after the procedure, infections set in, which required me to remain in the hospital for another week. It was an absolute nightmare.

My own complicity in this matter filled me with guilt from the moment I first saw the result. From that day I determined to do my best to never again allow shame and embarrassment to ruin my life. That has been a continuing struggle, but it has made me a better person.

The consequence of my circumcision is that I went from being embarrassed by not being able to retract my foreskin to being embarrassed by having been circumcised. To get beyond that pain, I determined to rise above it: to project personal pride and confidence to help override the desperate despair that I felt.

Missing, of course, are the marvelous sexual sensations that I once experienced. Ejaculations which once occurred with such pleasure, now have to be forced from a reluctant penis, now missing its most sensitive nerve endings. That bit of remaining frenulum has been my only consolation, though it is not always easy to stimulate during intercourse. My partners have been rubbed raw with every attempt.

About twenty years ago I discovered foreskin restoration, and immediately began working at restoring my own foreskin. To get and give support to other men, I founded the local chapter of the National Organization of

Restoring Men (NORM).[104] Having learned the many advantages of being intact, members of our group also man circumcision information tables at public events such as the local Martin Luther King Civil Rights Day. Helping and educating others has become another method of coming to terms with our circumcisions. Having mothers bring their intact sons to our table five or six years after they spoke with us makes the many hours we put into the effort worth every minute and every hour.

During this period I also discovered the great resource of the Internet, which served to shed fresh light on the complex anatomy and functions of the foreskin. One discovery that made my journey to circumcision and back rather bittersweet was learning that men with my original condition—a tight foreskin that resisted or prevented retraction—can easily remedy the problem through simple stretching exercises. Today I help such men solve my problem without benefit of circumcision, and that effort, too, helps give me peace. Would that doctors had the wit and intelligence to learn the same lesson.

Roy
75 years
Arizona, USA
27 November 2013

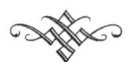

---

[104] The National Organization of Restoring Men (NORM) was founded in San Francisco in 1990.

Addicted To Rage And Sadness?

I read the TLC Tugger[105] page when I was fourteen and freaked the hell out and actually blacked out and I remember suppressing the memory deep inside. See, I had a great relationship with my parents at the time and the thought that they did something so fucked up was too much for me. I think I knew it would hurt our relationship if I let it in my head. I was also, as any fourteen year old, completely obsessed with sex and also a virgin. So the thought of not being able to fully enjoy the thing I wanted so much was also too hard to process. I was very emotionally immature at that age, I will admit.

So, fast forward to sixteen and I honestly didn't remember reading the TLC Tugger page. I had a girlfriend and was more worried about the game of trying to lose my virginity than anything else. Finally it happened. And nothing. I was wearing a condom and didn't feel anything. I barely stayed hard and never orgasmed. I dated the girl for two years and had tons of sex. She was a nympho and I learned how to get off better. She had to finish me by hand at least seventy-five percent of the time, though, and I couldn't feel anything with oral. I never really thought about why—I guess I was just too excited to be having so much sex to worry.

So, I had another girlfriend after that and she took birth control and so I didn't wear condoms. I could feel a little but not much. Something was still missing. It took me about thirty minutes to get off from intercourse without a condom.

Then I had a yearlong period of no sex and stumbled on circumcision topics again. It all came back. I feel like I went into a two-month psychotic breakdown. It destroyed me. It showed me how emotionally weak I am and showed me how scared and pathetic I am when I can't run to my parents' side for support. I felt like the best part of me is forever gone, and everyone around me will tell me I'm foolish for wanting my foreskin. I never attempted suicide or self-harmed, but did many things I regret and don't remember much from the last few months.

Recently, though, the fog seems to have cleared a bit and I'm not as furious at my parents anymore and I'm starting to be able to enjoy some things like playing the drums again.

---

[105] TLC Tugger is a foreskin restoration device made by TLCTugger.com.

I started restoration about a month ago and have had good results so far. I got a random blowjob and was actually able to orgasm from it. Even so, it did take a long time and she was the best oral I've ever had.

But anyways, I've been feeling a bit less psychotic lately and then tonight my band mate had his sisters and brother-in-law over and we had a great time. I felt happier then than I have in the last three years at least, partly because I feel like I'm falling in love with one of his sisters and just how well everyone got along.

But you know what? After everyone left, it was like I couldn't stand the feeling of being happy. I fucking just got out my phone and started reading about circumcision again and read topics that had women arguing in favor of mutilation and got myself all worked up again. Happiness was pretty much covered up by the rage and despair. And it's like I did it to myself on purpose. What the fuck is that shit? Does that make me a worthless person?

I know how bad circumcision is. I'm not discounting that at all, but I shouldn't let it keep me from being happy. I should be happy just to spite it, if anything. So why sabotage myself?

Greg
20 years
Nebraska, USA
25 November 2013

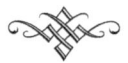

Adult Circumcision Trauma

I noticed lumps at the very most end of my foreskin that concerned me. The MD looked at the lumps and told me to go see a urologist, so I did. I saw a few, and they all suggested circumcision. That was not an option for me. Lumps persisted. Finally I saw a urologist in the area that told me he would biopsy the lumps, so at the very least they wouldn't bother me, and he told me that my wish of keeping the foreskin fully intact where the glans would be covered at all times will be honored.

This monster lied to me, however. I received an incredibly tight cut. Every cell of frenulum and inner tissue was gone. It was so tight I eventually had to have surgery to reshape the underside of the shaft skin. The mental trauma was so great I soon began self-cutting and by 2002, I was drinking and getting high every day. (I have been sober four years now, but still cut sometimes.) My girlfriend of many years couldn't deal with me and she left. I started dating another girl who thought I was fucked in the head and she also left. Now I can't have a simple relationship with any girl, even when sex is not involved—and it never is, because I feel completely defective.

I did find a lawyer. He opened my eyes to some real fucked up shit. I won't get into it, but it made matters even worse. We had a very solid case. I had written a note and my lawyer found it when he got the records. I made clear in the letter that Dr. Rapist was to only do a biopsy, no circumcision. (I guess in the horror of the situation I forgot about the letter.) The lawyer had a solid case for me. For whatever reason a medical examiner had to review the case. He must have been a monster as well because he didn't see cause for the case. I might be wrong but that's what I thought lawyers and judges were for. The legal system is a total joke in this country. Fucking Christ. The statute of limitations ran out before the matter got solved. Wouldn't you fucking know it!

I can't get on with my life now.

Hatelife
41 years
Minnesota, USA
18 September 2013

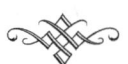

Baby Abuse, Adult Anger

Everybody knows that circumcision is horseshit. They won't circumcise themselves, but they won't hesitate or feel remorse when they do it to others. And since most circumcisions are performed on babies, due to the fact that they can't beat the holy hell out of the doctor, that's just bullying—hurting someone smaller than you just because you have the power to.

And since all bullies deep down are cowards, does that mean that every circumciser in the world is a coward? I almost take this as a compliment. Why couldn't they wait until I reached twenty-five years old to circumcise me? Is it because I'm too strong, too smart, and too good of a person for you, so that the only chance you have of hurting me is when I'm a defenseless fucking four-day-old infant? If child abuse is viewed as horrible and disgusting, then how do you picture baby abuse?

If it's not okay to circumcise anybody else, then why is it okay to circumcise me?

Circumcision doesn't just take away from you physically, but emotionally, psychologically, and even spiritually. As long as you keep telling yourself to accept what happened and do nothing but turn the page, you'll always be living a lie and you'll always be miserable. And lying about your feelings is the worst thing you can do.

We will work on the physical aspect. But the emotional aspect is even harder and is the hardest part of all, because our sacred emotional relationships hang in the balance of someone else's hands. Someone other than ourselves. That's why a lot of people have no self-worth today. They don't know how or can't get started. They make the same fucking mistake over and over again either because they're stupid or they're trapped. To build self-worth, it's always the same answer to any case: YOU NEED TO STAY AWAY FROM ASSHOLES!

On one hand, you have men who were intact at birth who got circumcised later on as an adult, who don't complain about sexual problems like sensitivity and stuff. Does it give encouraging news that being circumcised isn't that bad?

On the other hand, if restored men (who were circumcised at birth) are all saying that years of restoration turned their lives around both physically and mentally, than how could anyone keep endorsing this destructive procedure? Regardless of the divided opinions, one thing remains fact: If you circumcise your baby, you are taking a stupid and unnecessary risk. You are throwing your baby through a ring of fire, and you're hoping he goes straight through the loop without getting burned. We can all agree that's 100% fucked up.

Finally, as a circumcised and intelligent grown man capable of critical thinking, if I had the choice, rather than be circumcised—I'd actually choose the ring of fire.

CircVictim
28 years
Quebec, Canada
September - November 2013

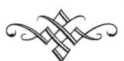

Circumcision Autobiography

I first realized I was circumcised at about age seven when I noticed the other boys in my class were different to me. I asked Mum about it, and her reply was "you have had a small operation." I didn't get much more information about it. In the change room they would run around with nothing on, but I could never do that because they might see how I was different. I would just change as fast as I could so I didn't get seen.

We moved house and my neighbor became my best friend. He was a little older than me. We used to play in the golf course which our houses backed onto. We would go to the toilet together, and play with our line of urine, height or distance, target shooting competitions. He was uncut, but would retract his foreskin to pee. I thought he had the same operation I had. One day I saw him retract his foreskin exposing his shiny glans. This was the coolest trick I'd ever seen, and this "operation" prevented me from being able to do this like him.

I went to school and compared or questioned other boys about this cool trick and asked if theirs did that too, and got most of them to show me. I wanted mine to be like theirs, where you could turn it inside out and make it look different. I could roll my skin over but it would roll back as soon as I let it go. Sticky plasters were my choice to hold the skin forward hoping it would grow back. But at seven years old I had no idea how to tape it correctly and used lots of band-aids. Thinking I might get told off, I hid the wrappers in my bedroom behind my washing basket.

Well, Mum found them and asked where I had hurt myself. I was ashamed to tell her what I was doing so I said nothing, but she knew something was up and went to my schoolteacher, thinking I was being bullied. I didn't know this, and carried on through the boys in the class showing me how their foreskin worked. Until one day one of the boys complained about it to the teacher, and then she took action. She asked the whole class who I had asked to see their privates. Boy after boy would yell out what I had been doing to them, and it turned out to be a "let it all out" session against me! I have never so embarrassed or ashamed in all my life to hear another boy say "he's circumcised and doesn't have a foreskin." My secret was out—the whole class knew—even the girls! Reduced to tears, I couldn't do anything. The teacher split the class and instructed just the boys about circumcision, and how either way is normal. After class she pulled me aside and asked about the band-aids.

Life carried on as usual for a few years. I accepted that I was the only circumcised boy in the class, when a classmate got the chop at about nine. He was absent for a few days. Returning, he confidently told us what surgery he had done.

I started puberty earlier than my peers, making me shy about my appearance during change room times. I would like to know if circumcision affects the onset of puberty.

I attended an all boys' high school, and the change room was full of pubescent boys so they all covered up. But from what I know not many of them were cut. Towards the end of school, losing our virginity was a big deal. My uncut friends had got there, and I lagged behind, and I thought this was due to being cut. Maybe girls could sense it. My friend told me he was cut. I was amazed to hear a friend I'd known throughout high school was cut, too. I didn't believe him. But, he also managed to have sex.

Before I started working, I used to hang at friends often for sleepovers, with girls and guys. None of these friends knew that I was cut. During a late night truth or dare, a girl asked cut or uncut? I was second to answer, I'd never told anyone since that day at primary school. I weakly replied, "Yes, I'm circumcised," expecting pointing fingers and laughter, but no. I got questions from the circle. What's it like? What's the difference? Really? When? Why? Shy me had all these questions about something I'd kept secret all these years. I gave answers and information to them—they were really interested. This built my confidence about myself. One girl's comment was "You're a dying breed." I used this quote for years whenever I was explaining about circumcision.

When I first had sex with my girlfriend, we had never seen each other naked or played around, as I was shy and didn't feel confident. When we had sex I felt nothing. It took about six or so sex sessions before I had trained myself to orgasm using my lack of sensitivity. I held out for ages about telling her I was circumcised, until I just had to tell her, thinking she would dump me for it. She knew nothing was any different, and we had showered and seen each other naked lots. I had to explain the difference between cut and uncut—she thought that's how men looked after puberty. Boys were covered. She shared this with her friends, that I was cut, and it was like an attractant to girls. I was rare, not your common guy. This made me lose my shyness. Girls wanted to try me.

I have got lots of compliments from the girls I have been with about my cut penis. It's cleaner, doesn't smell, feels harder. Some have just explored and admired my scar. But they don't know what I'm missing. The constant need for lube is probably the most annoying. Drying out and chafing is bad. Losing feeling or not being able to feel what a girl is doing, especially during oral, is the worst part, to the point that I have lost an erection due to no stimulation. Having little feeling means little control. I've had girls dry up, and I can't feel it, causing them to bleed.

Once I realized I was missing out, I started to talk to guys about the effects of circumcision. Most were unhelpful because they were intact. So I dropped the subject and enjoyed being cut. I could never talk to my parents about this kind of stuff, because they were too straight up about life and embarrassed to discuss sexual issues. Dad would just brush it away with some smart answer; Mum came across as being uncomfortable talking about it.

My old flat mate was a male model, and was getting my opinion on his latest shoot, he flicked through the decent photos and there was a nude picture at the end. He was very apologetic that he had made me see that, my only comment was, "You're circumcised?" I told him I was too. I then queried him about his nude modeling and being cut, as I'd never seen a cut model. We had a good chat about circumcision: We both didn't enjoy being cut but had grown to live with it. I mentioned that I heard a circumcision reversal on a TV drama show, and maybe he should look at getting it.

Thinking sewing skin on was as easy as cutting it off, he informed me that it takes years and he didn't want to do it. Curious, I asked him more about this reversal thing, and he told me about restoration by stretching. I didn't think much of it after he told me how long it takes, so I forgot about it.

A recent girlfriend was asking about my scar, and it was then she mentioned about getting my foreskin back. It came up after we got talking about her pre-school son being intact, he had showered with me and retracted his foreskin back to wash under it. I hadn't seen a foreskin retract in front of me in 20 years and it brought back the memory of how cool that trick was and how I wanted to be normal again.

I googled my new interest and found out about it. I read and studied devices. With my new wisdom I began my restoration. I started manually stretching and using tape properly, which I wish I had known back with the band-aids. I then moved on to a retainer which I made out of a kids' bubble tube and a mouthwash bottle cap. This device caused pinching of the skin and was hard to wear. I continued my study into devices and came up with a silicon bottle cap design, but the caps were too tight and cut off circulation.

Frustrated, I looked further into my design and come up with a bolt with silicon caps. Hoping to use the bolt as weight and silicon for comfort, yes, I achieved that, but it became time consuming during toilet calls. I then drilled a 5 mm (0.2 inch) hole through the bolt to allow urination. My device was comfortable and practicable. With no results, only sensitivity of the glans, I'd realized I had only made a retainer. Getting the kids' bubble tube, I filled it with lead with a nut cast in the top so I could screw onto the bolt retainer. I had created a retainer with a removable weight, capable of 24 hours constant wear. Having a weight jingling around your leg didn't suit my active lifestyle. It kept falling off.

I lost a weight one day while playing soccer with my daughter, and a few weeks later it turned up sitting on the fence post, I smiled knowing it meant nothing to anyone but me. I had already re-made another weight, so I left it on the fence post. I got over the weighted device and changed it to a push-pull by putting a rod through the bolt hole. It has a pusher plate that goes against the glans. The other end has a wedge screwed on, to which I attach a hair tie to apply constant pressure. This device is comfortable, compact, and I can wear it all day long while working, running, gym, or anything life has to offer.

Mike
28 years
New Zealand
20 November 2013

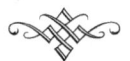

Circumcision Is A Cruel Hoax

I was born in Scotland in 1955. Like increasing numbers of men, I certainly appreciate the opportunity to discuss how upset I am to have been circumcised.

One unsettling aspect for me is that Britain's National Health Service stopped covering circumcision in about 1950. So my parents paid out of their own pockets to have me circumcised. The Royals were circumcised and I believe it was a status symbol. A status symbol? So what was the thinking there? That someone would look at me naked one day, see I am circumcised, and say there is a boy or man of status? What a ridiculous idea!

As a young man, I moved to the United States where, at the time, the circumcision rate was about ninety percent, and higher among Caucasians. It took a long time for me to realize that I was circumcised. The first hint was discomfort walking around as a young man. Circumcision exposes the glans and it rubs against clothing and is quite unpleasant. So much for the claim by American medical associations that the glans has no feeling.[106]

Then in college in the locker room I noticed that some men's penises look different and larger (they are larger), but still I didn't realize that they had a normal penis while I had a surgically altered one. Many boys were circumcised to save them from the embarrassment of looking different in the locker room, another ridiculous idea. I was not embarrassed. Based on what I know now, I would have been angry.

I never heard anyone discuss circumcision until my son was born. A physician asked whether we wanted him circumcised. He didn't look at my son once: in retrospect, it was a sales pitch. The only good thing he had to say about the foreskin is that it covers the glans and protects it from infection during infancy. He didn't say circumcision was painful or that it had risks or that it might affect my son's sex life.

He said that parents have the right to make the circumcision decision for religious, cultural, or personal reasons, including whether the father wanted the son to look like him. Well, the son wouldn't look like the father whatever surgery was performed on him. And parental power cannot possibly extend to cutting off part of one's child. Can I punch my child in the nose for religious reasons? Take out his eye? Operate on him to make his ears look

---

[106] Most of the glans surface has protopathic nerve endings that detect painful rather than pleasurable sensations as William notes. (Henry Head, *Studies in Neurology*, Vol. 1 (London: Hodder & Stoughton, 1920), 277.)

like mine? Because my god told me so? Or just because I feel like it today? And parents have the right to circumcise their sons but not their daughters? That can't be true either.

In retrospect, physicians who circumcise put parents on the spot and don't tell them the truth. What's easier than taking candy from a child? Getting a circumcised father's consent to do the same to his son.

So I started to research circumcision and as I see it, it is a hoax. American medical associations claim that with anesthetics, circumcision pain is "well tolerated." That seems very unlikely. Circumcision is extremely painful, often anesthetics are not used, and even when they are, they just slightly reduce the pain. Basically, helpless infants only a few days old are skinned alive without anesthetics, something no adult would agree to for himself. It's barbaric.

It took a long time for me to watch a circumcision video, but when I did, it was obvious that the baby was suffering extreme pain. Plus, babies must be terrified. American medical associations wrote in 1999, "Behavioral changes include a cry pattern indicating distress." No, really? So, what would be the way to avoid that distress? The answer doesn't seem to have occurred to many physicians.

Then I realized, that happened to me. Even though I don't remember it, I greatly resent that a physician, for a fee, strapped me to a board and cut off about half of the covering of my penis, probably without any anesthetic. What effect does that have on the infant brain? It can't be good. And I am upset with my parents for allowing it. What were they thinking? What did the doctor tell them? That it was good for my health? That's a lie. It hasn't improved my health. It has damaged my health.

In 1971 the American Academy of Pediatrics wrote: "The immediate hazards of circumcision of the newborn include local infection which may progress to septicemia, significant hemorrhage, and mutilation." In 1999, the American Medical Association wrote of terrible injuries that can result from circumcision which they called "untoward events."[107] The heartless bastards. Amputation of the penis and death are "untoward events?" "Madam, there has been an untoward event. Your son is dead. Sorry we forgot to tell you that could happen." At least I didn't have the glans of my penis cut off, or die from bleeding or infection like many other boys throughout history.

Today, American medical professionals claim that circumcision does not

---

[107] Council on Scientific Affairs. "Report 10: Neonatal circumcision" (Chicago: American Medical Association, 1999).

affect your sex life, but that is obviously untrue. The foreskin moves back and forth in a gliding action. Without a foreskin, that normal function is impossible. Ergo, circumcision destroys normal sexual function. The foreskin is full of nerves and blood vessels and highly erogenous. Studies show that it is the most sensitive part of the penis, more sensitive than any of the parts left after circumcision. This is only common sense. If the foreskin did not have any sensation, it would interfere with sex. American medical associations also acknowledged once that circumcised men masturbate more, so they know that it changes your sex life.[108] My guess is that circumcised men are perpetually horny because they are perpetually dissatisfied.

I know circumcision has impaired my sex life and for all of my adult life. I masturbate often, and although it is pleasurable, it is not completely satisfying. Nor is sex with women. So I believe it impairs marriages. As I got older, sometimes I could not reach orgasm, and would sometimes rub the shaft of my penis raw from trying, whereas the normal penis just folds and unfolds without friction, no lubrication required.

One day I saw online that in the erect intact penis, the foreskin spreads lubrication over the head of the penis. The circumcised penis by contrast is a dry stick. That was the moment I realized how much I had lost from not having a foreskin. I also realized that the impairment was getting worse with age.

Then I realized that circumcision is also bad for my wife. First of all, she has to work harder to bring me to orgasm, and secondly, the dry stick must be uncomfortable compared to the moist foreskin that glides with less friction.

About four years ago I learned about foreskin restoration, growing part of the foreskin back slowly over time. I started with no foreskin at all, or essentially none. After four years of continuous effort, the foreskin is beginning to reach and sometimes go over the corona or hump of the glans, called full flaccid coverage. It has been such an effort to put on and take off a device to stretch my foreskin for four years, I cannot tell you. I have to do this many times per day. And if I am somewhere in public, I have to find an enclosed toilet and do this next to people stinking up the stall next to me. Secondly, it will probably take me another four years to have erect coverage. Some unknown doctor hacked off my foreskin in a matter of minutes, and now I have to spend eight years to get just part of it back?

But foreskin restoration has greatly improved my sex life. That's what

---

[108] E.O. Laumann, C.M. Masi, E.W. Zuckerman, "Circumcision in the United States," *JAMA* 1997; 277(13): 1052-7.

everyone says who does it. In fact, I noticed improvement from the first few weeks. The glans of the circumcised penis is gray, and after covering it all the time, it becomes rosy in color and much more sensitive, in fact so sensitive that I have to cover the tip of the penis all the time; otherwise it feels like having sandpaper on it. Now the foreskin glides back and forth the way it is supposed to.

Sensation is much better even with only part of a foreskin. With the intact penis, the buildup of sexual tension and pleasure is slower. It's more controlled. With the circumcised penis, the internal shaft has become external. It did not evolve to function that way. I have read that the frenulum, often called the man's G-spot, also plays a role in ejaculation. I feel so sorry for men who don't have a frenulum.

In my opinion, orgasms are very weak circumcised, and greatly improved by foreskin restoration. This is even though I am only about halfway done, and will never have a complete foreskin with its ridged band, Meissner's corpuscles, Dartos muscle,[109] and full frenulum. I am guessing that sex is about half as good for me now as it should be, and that when I am done restoring, I will have about seventy percent of normal function back. I suspect that intact men have full body orgasms like women.[110]

To summarize, the American public has no idea what circumcision is about, because physicians who circumcise keep them in the dark. They get paid to do this, they have a trade association to promote circumcision, and they are never going to give it up until they are thrown in jail. Physicians don't tell parents that circumcision is painful, that it requires tearing the foreskin away from the glans, that anesthesia may not be used or does not work well, that it risks serious injury and death, that it harms all boys and men (i.e. unnecessary surgery is harm), and that it messes up their sex lives and that of their partners.

Physicians who circumcise and American medical associations also claim benefits where none exist. They claim that it prevents or reduces the risk of urinary tract infections, penile cancer, and STDs, including HIV. It's all a scare tactic. Circumcision doesn't prevent those diseases. Doctors don't make the difference clear. It hasn't even been proven that circumcision

---

[109] The Dartos muscle is a layer of smooth muscle within the penile and scrotal skin that contracts in response to low temperatures.

[110] Kinsey et al. indicate that about seventy-five percent of intact men have an orgasm that is more than urethral contractions alone, the common experience of circumcised men. (A.C. Kinsey, W.B. Pomeroy and C.E Martin, *Sexual Behavior in the Human Male* (Philadelphia: W.B. Saunders, 1948): 160-1.)

reduces the risk of penile cancer or STDs, including HIV. Even if it were true, those are rare diseases that can be avoided by washing one's penis (which presumably all men are happy to do), and by avoiding having sex with infected women or by using a condom. Thus, few boys or men benefit from circumcision at all. Only the most irresponsible do and probably only for a short time. Circumcised or not, men who have unprotected sex enough times are going to get STDs.

We are supposed to trust physicians. Their duty is to the patient alone. American physicians have knowingly misled parents since the 1800's. This is a huge blot on the medical profession.

For my part, I feel that I was robbed. I'm angry at my parents and the physician who circumcised me. I hate physicians who circumcise and their medical associations—they just lie about it and get away with it. I can't believe that a physician, who is sworn to improve health and to do no harm, could possibly do this to a helpless infant. If I were a physician, I would not cut off part of a boy's body for all the money in the world.

I have foreskin envy. Although I am able to deal with it, in part by doing something about it (foreskin restoration), I am extremely upset to have been circumcised against my will. I agree with European medical associations that there is no medical justification for this antiquated practice, it is unethical, and it violates the rights of the child. It saddens me to think that more than one million boys are still circumcised and harmed every year in the United States alone by their parents, all for no benefit at all, other than for physicians, who are supposed to improve the health of boys and men, not take it away. I'm looking forward to the day when physicians are held liable for non-therapeutic circumcision, as a court found in Germany, and put in jail where they belong.

William
58 years
Colorado, USA
24 November 2013

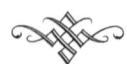

Circumcision, Judaism, And Choice

I am a Jewish man, and I grew up Orthodox. I was circumcised at eight days old, without anesthetic, and had *metzizah b'peh* (ritual oral suction) performed on me.

I will not divulge the present status of my religious observance, due to potential discrimination from one way or the other. However, I will state that for the vast majority of my life, I have been religious, and I still identify as a Jew and am proud to be one. I live in a Jewish house, in a Jewish community, and nearly all of my friends are Jewish.

I have also always had problems with my penis, but never once connected them to circumcision. Tight skin, painful erections, and tearing have frequently plagued me.[111] I even visited a doctor about the problems when I was younger; he said surgery was the only viable option, but he didn't recommend it, as it could make the issues worse. The doctor also informed me that the issues were probably due to circumcision, and I remember shrugging it off as simple bad luck on my part.

To me, circumcision was just something "everybody did," whether Jewish or not. It was not an invasive procedure, but a way of life. The doctor might as well have told me I was born with those issues, and it would have had the same effect on me as telling me it was from circumcision.

I remember the first time I ever saw an uncircumcised penis. My family was vacationing in Scandinavia when I was fourteen, and we were at a spa with a changing room. Almost everybody I saw was uncircumcised, and I had no

---

[111] Ancient Jewish circumcision (*bris/brit milah*) 'severed the frontal part of the foreskin' only, which was sufficient at the time to fulfill the religious requirement. During the first or second centuries CE, because Hellenized Jews were stretching their foreskins to be more acceptable to the Greeks, the rabbis reacted by introducing the more damaging *peri'ah* ('opening' or 'uncovering'). This involved "grasping the remaining foreskin and underlying mucosal tissue, forcibly separating this from the glans (using sharpened thumbnails), and tearing it away. Failure to remove all 'shreds' of foreskin tissue, the rabbis ruled, rendered the circumcision invalid." *Metsitsah* ("sucking") was probably introduced at this time to manage "the abundant blood flow" caused by the *peri'ah*. (Leonard B. Glick, *Marked in Your Flesh: Circumcision from Ancient Judea to Modern America* (York: Oxford University Press, 2005), 44-5). Post-Hellenistic or modern Jewish circumcision removes a large amount of tissue (as does American neonatal circumcision) and this explains Yechiel's erection problems.

idea why their penises looked the way they did. I wouldn't think about that incident again for years.

For me growing up, circumcision was never really discussed. I always knew what it was and was always aware of it, but to me, not doing it was never even an option. A couple of friends and I went through a brief rebellious stage where we doubted G-d's existence and questioned the religious aspects of Judaism from the inside out. We reassessed every single topic we had ever learned in school and by ourselves, and discussed the most minute details and problems in incredible depth. Not once did we ever bring up circumcision. It was something not even the most doubting of Jews questioned.

I had a roommate in college who was uncircumcised, from a country where the practice was not prevalent. He was just as curious about my circumcision as I was about his foreskin, and we often talked about the topic. However, this was mostly regulated to jokes and lighthearted remarks. I never once felt jealous of him or upset about my own circumcision, and simply thought his penis was different to mine, just as his skin color was.

Not too long ago, I was just aimlessly browsing the Internet, and began reading about the sexual effects of circumcision. The more I read, the more I began to realize that there are no good medical reasons for performing it indiscriminately, and the actual requirement for the procedure is rare. I was shocked. While I recognized that it was done to me with religious intent, I had always assumed it was medically beneficial as well, which is why there were non-Jews who would do it also, especially in the United States.

I talked to various people about it, and was disturbed by the vociferous defense of the practice. Jews obviously support it as a religious freedom, but I was surprised to see completely secular people and medical professionals defending it as well.

I was even surprised to see people who strongly oppose female genital mutilation dismiss male circumcision as "incomparable in any way." I think that whatever one's views on the respective severity of the procedures, they are most certainly comparable: They are rooted in religion and culture, they involve the slicing of the genitals, they are most often done without consent of the participant, and they are often propagated by people who have had it done to them.

It seemed to me that the only real defense people had for the practice was some inherent cultural or religious right. While I respect all religions, I realize that specific practices and beliefs are, and ought to be, prohibited. In the United States, the will of a Christian Scientist parent refusing medicine for his sick child must be overridden. A Jehovah's Witness may try and refuse a blood transfusion for his child, but a doctor is able to intervene if there is a threat to the child's life. Rastafarians are prohibited from smoking marijuana religiously, which doesn't hurt anybody. Those minority Shi'a Muslims who wish to draw blood from their children for the festival of Ashura are prohibited from doing so. Clearly, even in the religiously tolerant society of the United States, religious beliefs do not take precedence over common sense and child welfare.

The thing that struck me as bizarre was how quick non-religious people would be to defend infant circumcision. People seemed not to understand the idea that a circumcision is not something you can remove when you are older, but a foreskin is something you can remove if you do not want one.

The preventive measures I heard for doing it to babies were flimsy: Penile cancer is extraordinarily rare (in fact, less frequent than the most conservative estimates of complications from circumcision) and not a good justification at all and urinary tract infections are minor issues, and actually much more common in baby girls than baby boys. The main argument people told me was prevention of sexual disease, which is, of course, far less effective than safe sex and not an attractive proposition at that. Babies are not sexually active. When they reach the age where they begin to have sex, they can decide for themselves whether they would like a circumcision.

I do not oppose circumcision. I oppose circumcision for infants, because they do not have a say in the matter. An adult is free to choose what he wants to do with his body, but he shouldn't be free to choose what to do with someone else's. Had I been left uncircumcised and presented with the arguments as they are now, I would have never chosen circumcision for myself. Someone else may feel differently. That is his choice. But it is no one else's. It is difficult for me to reconcile my belief with my upbringing, but Judaism is a progressive religion.

I have encountered a decent amount of anti-Semitism within the intactivist movement, both from people who know I am Jewish and from those who do not. I will not deny that there are anti-Semites in the movement, and that some of it is anti-Semitically motivated. Nonetheless, there are anti-Semites and anti-Semitic motivations for members in the Republican Party, the Democratic Party, capitalists, anti-capitalists, communists, anti-communists, animal rights movements, environmental movements, and pretty much any social or political cause.

Accordingly, I do not think the intactivist movement itself is motivated by anti-Semitism. Anti-Semites and people who think that Jews are "barbaric" should realize that Jews compromise only 0.2% of the world, so stopping their circumcision won't really affect any global or national circumcision rate. In fact, if every Jew on the planet ceased circumcision today, it would have virtually no impact.

Additionally, complication rates for mohels (Jewish ritual circumcisers) are actually lower than those for medical doctors, since mohels specialize in what they do.[112] Doctors are also financially motivated, at least in the USA, and almost all mohels will perform the service for free if a family cannot afford it. Were I to choose to get circumcised, I would go to a mohel before a doctor.

This being said, I do recognize the fears of anti-Semitism felt by my fellow Jews. Anti-circumcision movements have indeed historically been enacted solely to target Jews, as only Jews practiced circumcision in those countries at the time. The Greek king Antiochus IV (c. 215 BCE–164 BCE) forbad circumcision in an effort to undermine Judaism, as did the Roman Emperor Hadrian (76 CE–138 CE), and many other rulers. Anti-circumcision advocates in the Middle Ages even forbade consensual adult circumcision for any reason. In those days, the only people who circumcised in the Western world were Jews, so targeting circumcision almost always meant targeting Jews.[113]

There can be no doubt that anti-circumcision promotion was once historically done to discourage the practice of Judaism. Today, however, most people in the Western world who are circumcised are, in fact, not Jewish. It is for this reason I do not view that vast majority of present day anti-circumcision as anti-Semitic. An anti-Semitic approach would simply call for ending *bris milah* (Jewish ritual circumcision) as opposed to the practice as a whole. It could more easily accomplish this as well, since most mohels are not doctors—despite the lower complication rate—and are performing medical procedures.

---

[112]An Israeli study of 19,478 boys found "no significant difference in the type of complications between medical and ritual circumcisions." The complication rate was low (0.34%), but the study of necessity excluded any adult complications such as the 'painful erections, and tearing' described by Yechiel. See Chaim J. Ben et al., "Complications of circumcision in Israel: a one year multicenter survey," *The Israel Medical Association Journal*, 7, 6 (2005): 368-70.

[113] For more on the history of circumcision in Judaism see Leonard B. Glick, *Marked in Your Flesh: Circumcision from Ancient Judea to Modern America* (York: Oxford University Press, 2005).

I think it is important for everyone, both Jewish and non-Jewish, to understand that Judaism is not a circumcision culture, but rather, it is a culture that happens to circumcise. Jewish adults should be free to be circumcised if they wish, and I myself predict that a very large percentage of them will choose to do so if and when infant circumcision is restricted. But it is important that we do not assume that everyone would make this same choice.

I did not ask for my circumcision or the problems it brought me, and I likely would not have chosen it as an adult. Again, others may feel differently. The issue is that the forcing a circumcision leaves no room for reversal, whereas forcing a non-circumcision can always be undone.[114] I think everyone should have the right to not have a procedure done to them that they do not wish to have. I think everyone should have the right to decide what they want to do with their body.

Yechiel
25 years
New York, USA
16 November 2013

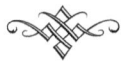

---

[114] This is the Open Future Principle, proposed by legal philosopher Joel Feinberg. See J. Feinberg, "The child's right to an open future," in *Freedom and Fulfillment: Philosophical Essays* (Princeton, Princeton University Press, 1992).

Conversation With My Dad

I was circumcised at birth and learned about circumcision at a very young age (of eight to ten years), first, when seeing my younger brother's intact penis during diaper changes, and again, when I found the word "circumcision" and asked my mother about it. I am the only cut male in my family. I guess that's the price I paid for being the firstborn son. My father, brothers and nephews are all intact.

I have always envied intact guys and their foreskins. I always wondered what it would look and feel like to have a foreskin of my own. I dwelled on this thought constantly. I realized that I would leave this earth and never know what I missed out on because of the ignorance of the doctors and nurses and the misinformation they fed my parents. Whenever I think about what was done to me and what continues to be done to boys around the world, it angers and depresses me.

I finally got a response from my dad about who made the decision to circumcise me and why. It doesn't make me feel too much better but it does give me peace of mind. So, I don't have to spend eternity wondering. Now the healing begins.

Dad's Reply:

Hello My Son. Hope everything is going well for you. Well. To begin on the subject of circumcision, back in the 1970's there were a lot of awful things going on, like syphilis, gonorrhea and tightness of the foreskin, which is painful enough. I really wish it was done to me, but I actually thought that it would be a good thing to do, as far as the protection from all the diseases that were easily caught back then. Forgive me for making that decision for you at the time; I really meant for it to protect you, not hurt! It was a very scary thing to have back then believe me, very scary. Again my apologies! I Love You and Miss You and I hope we can someday see past this medical procedure that was done to you and millions of adults and children around the world, just for protection from all easily caught diseases known to man. I'm still wary about what can be caught and what can't be caught, but one thing I know for sure is that having the foreskin is much more at risk to getting a venereal disease than having circumcision. I really hope that this will help you in your debate about the reason why it is done. Love you. Let me know if this was reason enough or not!!!

Son's Response:

Hey Dad. I'm glad you are doing OK. It's good to hear from you. Thanks for getting back to me. I almost forgot I sent that message. I appreciate your honesty with me, and sharing why you thought it was best to have it done to me, even though I disagree with it. As much as I hate being circumcised (I won't go into the reasons right now) I do forgive you. I have always wondered why it was done to me and who ultimately made the choice and now I know. Thank you.

Did you know that outside of the USA circumcisions of males are very rare? The US has the highest rate of circumcision and the highest rate of STDs, AIDS and HIV in the western world. Sexually transmitted diseases have nothing to do with an infant's penis. Almost every male I know is intact, except for maybe two or three. And none of them have had any issues. In the end it should be the Adult Man's choice as to whether he would want a surgical procedure done on his most private body part and only when he is old enough to make that decision for himself.

If you'd like to learn more there are a number of good Internet sites.

Thanks dad. Love you and miss you.

Mikey
37 years
New Jersey, USA
3 October 2011

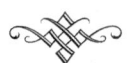

Conversations With My Sons

I, too, am cut. But I have never blamed my parents for taking away my foreskin. Yes, I wish it had not happened. But I am intelligent enough both cognitively and emotionally to believe and accept that they made a decision based on what they knew, and what the doctor recommended or persuaded them to do. It was not done with malice.

I have two sons and the first one I had circumcised. I, too, was ill informed and naive about circumcision. I followed the logic I had been given: sons should look like their fathers, and the doctor knows best. That has changed, of course.

My one-day-old son was snuggled in my arms when the nurse came in and told me it was time to circumcise him. I handed him into her arms, she smiled and said, "I'll be right back." Moments later I heard my son screaming in pain and I thought I was going to die. I cried at that moment over the pain he was experiencing and I was helpless to remove it or protect him. I didn't want my wife to see me cry at such a wonderful time in our life, the birth of our first child. But I could not hide my emotions. She, too, was horrified to be able to hear his pain.

At the time, neither of us understood the procedure completely. I later began researching circumcision. My wife and I began discussing it often. Our decision was secure; if we had another son, he would not be circumcised. We did have another son and we battled the doctors on the issue. I won.

I am now restoring my foreskin. My sons are in their twenties. I have a very supportive wife. Recently I talked with my sons about my journey toward restoring my foreskin. It was an opportunity to present the facts surrounding the issue. They listened intently. I did not know how they would respond to their Dad doing such a thing. We have a very good relationship, but this was something out of the ordinary for their Dad to do!

I sincerely apologized to my oldest son for having him circumcised. He looked me in the eyes and told me he was not angry or upset. He loved me. Now he is interested in restoring. Who knows? We may be restoring our foreskins at the same time. My youngest son just smiled and said, "Thanks, Dad, for leaving me with a foreskin. I wish you and my brother had one, too."

I have spent their lifetime nurturing our open, honest, and loving relationship. I know not everyone has that kind of connection with their sons. Sons need their Dads and I wish those of you who have strained relationships could at least forgive them for taking away your foreskin. Perhaps they were acting out of ignorance and naïveté as I was and my parents were.

It has been a wonderful and freeing experience to start restoring my foreskin and to have had the conversation with my sons. Frankly, it has opened a new level of trust and openness for us.

It takes courage to forgive. It is not easy and sometimes it is a journey. Consider taking the first step.

Restore1
50 years
California, USA
4 March 2012

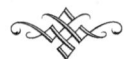

Crown Of Thorns

When I was seven and my brother was ten, my parents told us that there were these bad things in your throat called tonsils, and that normal people didn't have these bad organs, because they had them cut out, and only ignorant people who didn't know any better, and/or poor people who couldn't afford the surgery had tonsils.

I thought that was the stupidest bunch of nonsense I'd heard of. There was nothing wrong with my throat, and I did not need any surgery on my throat.

I'm sure I told my parents what I thought about the idea of a surgeon cutting part of my throat out, but at seven years old, I did not have any access to any medical journals to show my parents that tonsillectomy was, by that time, a discredited surgery and that it was no longer performed routinely. And, even if I could have made such arguments to my parents, it wouldn't have stopped them from committing the atrocities they did against the bodies of my brother and me.

My brother and I both begged our parents not to have this stupid, unnecessary surgery done to us. We were told that "we are adults, and cutting out part of children's throats is what we adults do to you children, and it doesn't matter what you think about it, or how you feel about it, it's going to be done to you and your brother."

I hated the very thought of someone cutting out part of my throat, and did not want part of my throat, or any other part of my body, cut off, or any other surgery done to me. Neither my brother nor I were sick, and what was done to us, was done as a "rite of passage." At that time I didn't even know that term, but that's what it was, and it was a "rite of passage" that neither one of us wanted any part of.

Neither my brother nor I were told that there was another cruel "rite of passage" that our parents planned to do to us, that was even more horrible than cutting out our tonsils, and I'm sure you know what that was. We did not find out about this "other" cruel thing our parents planned to do to us, unaware, until after we "came to" from the anesthetic.

This stupid act of cruelty that our parents did to both my brother and me is a trauma that has scarred me, haunting me to this very day with nightmares.

How any parent could treat their own children so cruelly is beyond me. It is such a horrible story I can tell but a little of it at a time.

Well, about a year or so after our parents told us that all normal people did not have tonsils, because they had been cut out, but not telling us that there was something that was also cut off of little boys, our parents apparently decided it was time to end the delay in doing their stupid, cruel, ritualistic "rites of passage" on their two sons.

We were taken to a surgeon who didn't really examine us, but the surgery was scheduled, sometime in early 1959. At that time, I was seven years old, and my brother ten years old.

Years later, after I finally got up the nerve to try to discuss it with my parents, my mother told me that the surgeon told them that he did not take out tonsils at the request of parents, and did so only on the recommendation of an examining doctor. My parents were friends of our "family" doctor, so he told the surgeon that my brother and I had had a lot of sore throats.

How I wish I had never told my parents when I did have a sore throat!

But they still would have done the two atrocities to my brother and me even if we had never complained of any sore throats.

The surgeon apparently accepted the family doctor's recommendation, which he undoubtedly gave just to stay friendly with my parents.

I suppose the surgeon was somewhat enlightened, but not enough, as far as taking out tonsils at the request of parents went, but he had no such qualms at all about cutting off part of my and my brother's penises at the request of our parents. He did not even examine our penises to see if there was anything wrong that required surgery.

After my parents told me what was going to be done to my brother and me (although they only told us HALF of what they were planning to do to us), I came to realize human beings, or at least some human beings were sadistic, although I had never even heard that word. I realized they had a desire to inflict pain and cruelty on others, and often did so in stupid "rites of passage," which I wanted no part of. I could not see why people wanted to be so mean.

And, when some other kid told me that having your tonsils cut out was a good thing because you get to eat ice cream, I thought, those kids are as stupid as the parents who do this atrocity to their children. I had eaten ice cream, and I sure as hell did not want to get to eat any ice cream, only one time in my life, by having my tonsils cut out.

I naturally knew it would be horribly painful, and it was.

I was so terrified of what my parents were going to do to me and my brother, that the morning of the scheduled surgery, I seriously considered running off and hiding in the wooded area around our residence, and that would stop their evil plans.

But, I was too scared to do so. As much as my brother and I feared and hated our parents forcing upon us having our tonsils cut out, we did not run away on the morning of the atrocity, but went on ahead to the hospital.

We both had a natural aversion to someone cutting out part of our throats, and if we had known what else our parents had planned for us, we certainly would also had a natural aversion to it, too.

Waking up from the anesthetic is a horror I will never forget and which has haunted me since 1959 and will haunt me until the day I die!

First thing I remember was a horrible, horrible pain in my throat, unlike any I have ever had, before or since. And, then I vomited blood! The nurses held out a turquoise plastic jar to catch the blood.

Then, I discovered that there was a Crown of Thorns around my penis!

I use those words because the only thing I had seen before was the paintings of the Crucifixion of Jesus, and the Crown of Thorns on his head.

That is exactly what the horrible, brown, scratchy stuff that was all around my penis head looked like. Another comparison might be a ring of barbed wire.

I immediately thought, what does this crown of thorns around my penis have to do with part of my throat being cut out?

Then, I realized it had nothing to do with cutting out part of my throat.

It was something else that our parents did not tell us about and, because it was so horrible, they wanted it done to us without our knowledge.

If, before the surgery, someone had told me that our parents would have part of my and my brother's penises cut off, I would have said, "No Way. Our parents would never do such a thing to us. They are cruel, and mean, and stupid to want our tonsils cut out, but they would never, ever think of having part of our private parts cut off!"

Well, waking up in that hospital to that horror I found out differently. Our parents had played a dirty, rotten, despicably evil trick on both my brother and me, and I knew that I could not trust them.

I was as angry as hell over what our parents had done to my brother and me.

First, they had the horrible pain inflicted on our throats. Then, just like the people who crucified Jesus, they enjoyed more sadistic delight by having us shamed and humiliated by having part of our penises cut off, and a crown of thorns put in our foreskins' place.

Once we came out from the anesthetic, our parents obviously couldn't keep the secret that they had had a second atrocity planned for us.

That morning in the hospital is the first time I recall hearing the word, "Circumcised." If I had heard it before, it went in one ear and out the other.

Our parents really fixed us up good!

By having our penis skinned and a horrible pain in our throats, my brother and I couldn't shout out at them: "WHAT THE HELL HAVE YOU DONE TO OUR PENISES ??? !!! You didn't tell us about this !!!"

No, we could barely speak; the pain in our throats was so horrible. Makes me think of vets who neuter dogs, then cutting the dog's vocal cords, so their cries of pain cannot be heard.

I don't remember being able to ask any questions, but do remember our father telling us, "You have been circumcised." And, he drew a picture to try to explain what had been done to us, but the drawing didn't mean anything to me.

My penis really didn't look any different after the cutting than it did before. The reason?

Mother told me that while my brother had been left intact, that my father had insisted on having me cut, when I was born three years later, despite the doctor not wanting to do it.

But, my penis had not been skinned to my father's satisfaction, so he wanted me skinned again, and that stupid, evil surgeon did it simply at my father's request.

I never remember my glans being covered with skin before that atrocity in the hospital, and it didn't seem that anything was missing afterwards, but I did know my penis had been cut, and that horrible, horrible crown of thorns put around it.

I was as angry as hell at my parents, the doctors, and everyone else who did this senselessly brutal act to my brother and me.

Ever since that morning in the hospital all those years ago, every time I hear any word starting with "cir-" spoken, I relive the horror I woke up to in that morning. "Circumstances," "circumference," any word that starts with those three letters, brings back all the horror to me.

My brother's crown of thorns hurt him so much, that, despite the pain in his throat, he let the nurses know it.

I did not know until years later, when my mother told me that during our first night at home after the atrocity, that the stitches came loose and my brother had to be taken back to the hospital to be re-stitched.

In my dying moments, I will relive the horror that was done to my brother and me in that hospital, as I have done every day of my life since.

Bill Sloan[115]
62 years
South Carolina, USA
18 September 2013

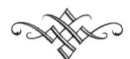

---

[115] This story is taken from oregonintactivist.com with permission of the author.

72

Disconnected

On the outside looking in, my life seems pretty damn good. I am good looking, successful in my career, and live in one of the best suburbs of Melbourne. I have plenty of friends and enjoy an active social life. But once you scratch beneath the surface, you will find a man who has been tormented his whole adult life by a botched circumcision.

The psychological trauma that I have suffered and continue to suffer is something I would wish on no other human being. Every single day of my life is consumed with the ongoing effects of what was done to me as an infant. It has shaped my experience of life and has left me a shattered man fighting suicidal thoughts.

I have just endured the breakdown of a relationship with a woman that I was falling deeply in love with. This is the woman that I want to marry. She is a beautiful blonde, blue-eyed, thirty-four-year-old air hostess, and she had said on numerous occasions that I was going to be the father of her children.

But she left me after five months.

We all know why she left.

I am now at the point sexually where I barely feel a thing during intercourse. I am on Viagra because I find it nearly impossible to keep an erection during sex, but having an erection really isn't that great when you still can't feel anything. You are basically just going through the motions and you remain firmly in your head and not in your body.

If I am disconnected from myself during sex, then you can be sure that I am disconnected from my partner. My ability to pleasure her becomes incredibly difficult when I am feeling very little pleasure myself.

My ability to ejaculate has been severely compromised. It was only on three occasions during our whole relationship that I managed to come.

So I can add this relationship to the incredibly long list of what my circumcision has cost me. Another chance at building a family and living a life with the woman I love has slipped through my fingers once again. The despair that has consumed me since she left has brought to the surface thirty years of pain, which began when I stared down at my penis as a teenager and wondered why it was covered in hair.

There was no Internet to do any research and I didn't know anything about circumcision. All I knew was that something was wrong.

My circumcision is so tight that I have what is known as *penoscrotal webbing*.[116] My scrotum is drawn up onto my shaft and I have hair that goes all the way up to the circumcision scar because all the skin of my penis was cut off.

My youth was consumed with my shame at how unattractive my penis was.

I would shave if I ever thought there was the chance of any intimacy, but if I was unshaven there was no way that I could let a girl see it. I was always petrified that she would feel the hair, or the stubble of hair once it started to regrow. Hands up: How many girls would like to date a guy with a hairy penis? Not many.

I have memories that carry immense regret.

Picture yourself with a beautiful girl on a deserted beach as the sun comes up on a new year. You have been kissing for hours and have just gone for a skinny dip. You sit on a log and she comes out of the water and lays herself across you.

Your mind is racing because you know that your penis is not prepared at all and you are in the middle of nowhere. There's no rushing to the bathroom to fix yourself up. You make some sort of lame excuse about getting back to the campsite. A moment that could have been etched into your brain as one of the most joyful has just been converted into its opposite.

Of course, you never hear from the girl again.

A party is getting out of control. Two girls grab you by the hand after they have just been kissing each other in front of you. They start to lead you towards a bathroom and your heart starts pounding, because your penis is covered in hair and you can't let them see it in this state. It would be far too embarrassing.

Again you offer some lame excuse and you are left to live the rest of your life wondering just what would have happened in that bathroom.

Beautiful experiences in life are turned on their head and left as eternal regrets because a person that I never met butchered my penis a day after I was born.

I have always struggled sexually during my relationships and never really knew why. I thought that the hair was an issue, but that once it was dealt

---

[116] *Penoscrotal webbing* is a complication of circumcision in which the skin of the scrotum is connected along underside of the penis for a greater distance than normal.

with, I was basically normal. But, in fact, my sensitivity has always been an issue, and, now that I have hit forty, it has become the major issue related to my botched circumcision.

I have just endured a year of getting laser hair removal on my penis (ouch) and I am happy with the results, although there are still hairs growing there. But, my level of sensitivity is now so low that I feel too bad to inflict myself on another partner.

Why on earth would she stick around if we can't have good sex?

I am even nearing the point of giving up completely, because I just had an immensely beautiful woman in my bed and I really didn't enjoy the experience that much. I was so stressed by the fact that I couldn't pleasure her or myself that there were only fleeting moments where I really let myself go. The despair I feel now is so overwhelming that I wonder if it was worth it at all.

That's why I have spent so many years of my life avoiding relationships. I would be single for years at a time, while my friends would all be scratching their heads wondering why I was not "getting out there."

The stress involved in being intimate was often so great that I chose to remain celibate. My most recent relationship has probably confirmed that I will go back to being single again. When I'm single I don't need to confront the fact that I am a failure as a man.

There is nothing more mysterious or beautiful than the connection between a man and a woman. And that is where circumcision hits hardest, stripping a man of his essence. Perhaps I am one of the more extreme cases, but every single man who has had his penis cut has had part of his essence stolen from him, whether he realizes it or not.

For society, religion, my parents, or anyone else to tell me that they have the right to hold me down when I am born and strip me of my masculinity, to strip me of my chance at joy, and then collectively shrug their shoulders when it all goes wrong has left me at the very edge of my sanity.

Every single moment is tainted by what happened to me. Past regrets, unfulfilled desires, tattered self-confidence, despairing of the future—the level of hopelessness that I feel now is complete.

My only thought is that I must do all I can to ensure that I save as many men from my fate as possible. If I can do that, then my life may very well have been worth it.

Gary
42 years
Australia
2 October 2013

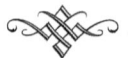

Finally Had The Discussion

Today, something in me wouldn't let me go one step further without finally having the circumcision discussion with my parents. I just couldn't function at all until I got everything I have been thinking and feeling out into the open.

For a long time I have been avoiding talking to them for pretty much any reason. I was too afraid of what I might say, or that I might be unable to contain myself if the wrong word slipped out. As they are two of the most important figures in my life, and my support network for virtually every other part of my life, I was afraid of damaging that relationship.

The problem is that keeping silent was eating me up inside. Anger was turning into a monster that was keeping me up at night, and keeping silent was feeding the anger inside of me.

It was a no-win situation for me. I didn't want to damage our relationship by accusing them of horrible deeds. They are really quite wonderful parents, but by keeping it all bottled up inside I was pulling away from them, and having less and less to do with them over time.

It was selfish of me, but I had to talk to them, or cut myself off from my parents completely. Either way, I would prefer them to know what was bothering me and attempt to repair the relationship with them, over never speaking to them again.

Without warning them what it was about, I called them on Skype video chat.

It was hard to bring up, but after the usual meaningless small talk I managed it. I started to ask them some basic questions about my circumcision as an infant. What day I was cut on, what was asked of them, if I had any complications. They were surprised, but answered honestly and simply. I learned that I was circumcised with a Plastibell device.[117] I had honestly thought I was cut with a Gomco Clamp[118] due to the type and amount of damage.

Then the hard part. They wanted to know why I was curious.

---

[117] The Plastibell is a circumcision device invented by Hollister Inc in 1950, consisting of a clear plastic ring with a deep circumferential groove.
[118] The Gomco Clamp is a circumcision device developed by Hiram S. ('Inch') Yellen and Aaron A. Goldstein and used in the USA from 1935.

I explained the issues I was dealing with. It was very difficult admitting these things to my parents and I was shaking. I explained the missing frenulum, the tight erections, the malapposition of the scar,[119] and the partial meatotomy I have.[120] The partial meatotomy came from either the doctor removing the frenulum and cutting too deeply, or cutting from the ventral side of the penis instead of the dorsal side when he split the foreskin from the head of the penis. In this process he likely nicked/split the urethral opening.

It was at this point that my mother started to get upset. They asked how I knew these things.

I then admitted to my foreskin restoration, and that since I have developed enough skin to cover the split in the lower part of the glans, I have managed to counteract the drying out of the meatus, and have finally eliminated the pain I have had while urinating. I went thirty-nine years thinking it was normal to feel a bit of pain while peeing (sometimes a lot), but that I finally didn't feel that way anymore.

It was at this point that my mother really started crying, and my father became really silent.

Mother: "What are we supposed to do about this now? It's not like we can go back in time and change anything."

Me: "It's not about going back in time. The past is the past. This is about changing the future. It is about making the future different."

Mother: "What are we supposed to do about it?"

Me: "Nothing, but be a sounding board for me if I need some support. Maybe tell the next person who asks that circumcision is a mistake. I'm the one dealing with this, and I need you both to know because not talking about this with you is killing me."

Mother: "How long have you felt this way? Have you always hated us?"

Me: "I've felt this way for a long time, but I've never hated you. I still don't hate you. I love you. But I am going through a lot, and I need the people I love the most to be in my corner, or I can't go on. I've been afraid to talk to you about this because I knew it would hurt you, and you don't deserve it. But not talking to you about this is torture, and it just makes me avoid you. I was cutting you out of my life because of this, and that's wrong. I was punishing you because of this, and you deserve to know why. Not having this

---

[119] *Malapposition* is the misalignment or two opposing bodily structures.
[120] *Meatotomy* is the enlarging of the urethral opening.

conversation was doing as much damage as having it. I love you both too much to punish you, and not even let you know why."

Mother: "What do you want us to do now?"

Me: "Hopefully, you'll be on my side. I may need you to answer some questions, or I might just need a sounding board. That's all I need from you."

My mother left the room about this point, and my father finally spoke to me.

Father: "I think you should probably get some help for this. I think you need to talk to somebody ... professionally."

Me: "I have, Dad. I still am. I'm part of a support group online, and I am getting help. I've been getting help for a lot longer than I have been talking to you about this. I'm talking to you, because you are my real life support network. You are the people I care most about, and without people who love me knowing, I just can't ever heal fully. I know you may not be unhappy about your own circumcision, but that doesn't mean I don't have the right to be unhappy about mine. I've suffered a lot thanks to it, and I just can't deal with it in the shadows anymore. I need to take this step to stay healthy. You may think I am angry with you, but I'm not. I just need you to know. I need you to be on my side. Can you do that?"

Father: "Of course I can."

The conversation went on for quite a long time after my mother returned. They questioned me quite a bit, and I explained that I had been researching the issues deeply for a long time. I told them that I was sorry that bringing up the subject had hurt them, but that I was thinking of the next generation. My nieces will soon be marrying and having children of their own, and my parents may one day be asked the circumcision question. I hoped that they would simply answer that I had been circumcised and that it was a mistake.

They told me that they wouldn't offer an opinion because circumcision is a "personal family choice."

I answered that I hoped they would offer an opinion and that it isn't a family penis or the parent's penis. The only one who owns the penis, and who has to deal with the consequences for the rest of his life is the child to whom the penis is attached.

My father came back with, "When I was in the hospital for my prostate, the old guy who I shared the room with had to get circumcised because he was having health issues and couldn't clean himself anymore."

His hospital roommate was in his late seventies.

I told them that is not a reason to cut a baby when he is just born. At least that old guy got to enjoy his entire body for seventy plus years before he was cut.

My dad looked visibly shaken by that statement. He went silent again at that point.

My mother then said that her father, who was intact (her brothers were all intact, too), had problems with his foreskin, and they didn't want me to suffer that.

I told her that just because one person has an illness is no guarantee that someone else will, too. I reiterated that I was circumcised, and have problems with my circumcision. He was not circumcised and had problems. Everyone is different, and one thing does not equal the other.

She started crying again.

The conversation went on quite a while, and I must have apologized to them dozens of times for hurting them by bringing this up so late into my life, but that I was only doing it because emotionally I felt I had no other choice, and that I hoped we could all become stronger because of it.

My mother cried a lot, and I know she blames herself. She repeated many times that she's always guessed I was harboring some sort of hatred or anger, but she could never understand what it was. She knew what it was now. She apologized to me.

My father was less understanding, but made a point of telling me he understood, and hoped he could help.

It was very emotional, and I told them I just wanted to be more open with them because they are wonderful parents, and I really need them in my life.

The conversation ended by my parents berating me for my various life choices thus far. I don't have a good enough job, I'm living in too expensive a city, no plan for my future, that sort of thing.

I let them go off on me. It's nothing I don't already tell myself a thousand times a day, and frankly they can't put much of a dent in the concerns I have for myself. I've always known how they feel, and it was a relief to hear them finally say it out loud.

It sounds like they were trying to get verbal revenge on me for making them feel bad, by trying to make me feel bad, but that's not what it was. I invited them to tell me what was really on their minds. It was part of my goal to get them to open up. It was a huge relief. Keeping things bottled up isn't healthy.

Not for me, and certainly not for my parents. I'm glad they did.

The conversation ended with all of us telling each other how much we loved one another, and plans for how we will get together in the future. By the end of it, tears of grief had transformed to tears of joy. Mine and theirs both.

I am very glad I had the courage to engage in this conversation. I feel like a giant weight has been lifted from my shoulders.

Tomorrow finally feels like a brighter day.

Canaanite
39 years
Canada
16 December 2013

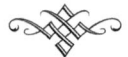

From Anger To Forgiveness

I struggled with grief and anger about being circumcised for over a decade. I carried a seething rage that would nearly boil over every time I heard the prefix "circ." I hated my parents and would likely have attacked the doctor who circumcised me had I come across him. Today, I am healed. I would like to share my story to encourage those who are still healing.

I learned what circumcision was from the Internet when I was about eleven or twelve. I had a loose circumcision, with most of my frenulum left and no apparent scar, so I chose to believe that I was not cut. In retrospect, I don't think I could've handled knowing that I was at that point. Around maybe thirteen or fourteen, I realized that I was indeed cut, at which point I chose denial and told myself it was a good thing.

I held on to that denial until I was seventeen, at which point I discovered foreskin restoration, along with details about all that I had lost. That's when the denial melted away and was replaced with fury I had never known before. Anger protected me from being overwhelmed by the grief, which at times had me contemplating suicide. Over time I learned to suppress the grief and anger to some extent, but it left me hypersensitive to anything related to circumcision and it did nothing to address the hatred.

I tried various restoration methods and kept giving up for various reasons. In my early twenties I finally started retaining[121] full time. I started at a Coverage Index (CI) 4 or 5, so I could retain from the start with o-rings, but problems with that method led me to use tape for years.[122]

At twenty-five, I finally discovered TLC Tugger[123] and ordered the whole set. I had issues using the Tugger and quickly gave up, but the Your Skin Cone[124] was like a dream come true for me, and I have been retaining 24/7 ever since. But the anger, grief, and hatred remained dormant, still poisoning my soul.

---

[121] *Retaining* refers to keeping the glans permanently covered.

[122] The Coverage Index is a classification system that gives numerical values to describe the length of foreskin; CI-1 means no foreskin (i.e. all has been removed by circumcision) and CI-10 means there is enough foreskin to overhang the top of the glans. See http://www.newforeskin.biz/.

[123] TLC Tugger is a foreskin restoration device made by TLCTugger.com.

[124] Your Skin Cone is a device manufactured by TLCTugger.com used to keep any remnant foreskin covering the glans to restore sensitivity.

I decided to start choosing to forgive. Whenever the feelings came up, I would mentally go through the list of everyone I forgive for my situation and then try to repress the feelings as quickly as I could, lying to myself that I was over the pain. That began my true healing, but I was still missing a couple of important steps.

Over the course of months and regular discussions about my feelings with my wife, I came to realize the problem with how I handled my pain. I tried to tell myself that I was over it in a futile attempt to alleviate it. When I finally accepted that I had been circumcised, that I had been robbed of the things we all wish we could get back, that it had hurt me to the core, and that I had been suffering for years as a result, it was like a veil was lifted.

Finally, the forgiveness was real. I accepted the pain and sorrow in its fullest and then I let it go. I could truly move on. The prefix "circ" lost its power over me. Circumcision now fills me with empathy. The word no longer stings.

The most joyous part of it all for me was that resentment was replaced with gratitude! I realized that I had given up so many times on so many restoration methods because the process put my circumcision in my face, reminding me of my pain, making it nearly impossible for me to suppress it. So I would give up and resume my suppression. It was an attitude of gratefulness that allowed me to begin restoring consistently. I am grateful that my circumcision was a loose one. I have nearly my entire frenulum and enough inner skin all around to almost cover my flaccid glans, though my scar line still rests on the inside of my foreskin at present. I'll probably never have spontaneous rollover, as my glans is quite prominent, even in my most flaccid state. But, I would say I started at a CI-4 or 5 as I could always stay consistently covered when flaccid. I'm also grateful that I seem to have no apparent scar; there is simply a line at which point my inner skin meets my outer skin, akin to a tan line.

However, even had my circumcision been much worse, I would still find gratitude in whatever I had left. For years I would be bothered by the thought that it must be nice to be a woman to be spared my mutilation, frustrated with and ashamed of my damaged member. Now I can finally appreciate my manhood and enjoy my penis, and I know I would even as a CI-0. I would be grateful just to have a penis, and I am incredibly grateful that I have discovered that it's possible to restore it.

Now I'm restoring daily, gratefully appreciating the process, along with the support for it that I can find on the Internet. I intend to restore until I can get an erection in any temperature or condition and maintain complete coverage without having to touch my foreskin. At present I have enough foreskin that it can hang over the edge of my corona with an erection while standing up (but it retracts if I lean back much), so I have several years of tugging to go, probably. But I am always grateful for the coming day when I will have finished restoring and completed my journey of healing.

J. Rook
28 years
Michigan, USA
12 December 2012

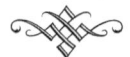

Foreskin Restoration Solved My Wife's Pain

Like many of us, I too was cut right after being born. My dad was intact but only at a Cl-5. I thought that when I grew up that I would be like him, since my cousins were all like me. Then around age ten I found out what really happened to me and figured it was just the way things were in these days. In my teenage years I noticed it took a lot of work to ejaculate and thought I must be doing something wrong because of the pain of being tight and not feeling much. Years went by and sex did not really appeal to me much, since I was working all the time, was poor, and did not think anyone would be interested in me, anyhow.

Then I met my wife. For the first few years, sex was good, but she complained that I was pounding so much and I tried to change. Then the worst thing happened. She began having a lot of pain during sex. We went to doctors looking for answers. Pelvic exercises, creams to numb, hymenectomy, water-based lubes, silicone lubes, etc., none seemed to help much at all. To add to the mess, my wife began drying out due to her hormone issues with her ovaries. We finally got to the point of going months without sex.

So I got tired of the whole thing and began looking about for what I could maybe do. That is when I found a website talking about how the foreskin helps during sex. I searched many sites and found out the concept of regrowing foreskin. I figured if she went through so much, I would try, even if it hurt for awhile. Then I found Paul's restoration site and began my journey with the pill canister.

Three years later finally I got to Cl-5 and my wife no longer has any pain. I sure wished I had found this information out when I was young, so I could have avoided all this from happening to me. I can't believe that after seeing all the doctors and others, no one talked about the foreskin. I guess there are a lot of people out there who don't really understand its purpose and what it can add to our lives.

Swampthing
49 years
Georgia, USA
27 February 2014

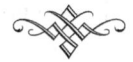

He Won't Remember It Anyway

I was raised in a family that didn't know how to talk about sex or our bodies. My parents even used made up words to talk about bathroom behaviors and body parts.

Though I was raised in this kind of family, I still had questions, but I had to learn not to ask them. I was very small when I started asking my mom about it. Of course nobody had ever mentioned it, but I knew that I had been "CUT" down there. I actually believed at the time that the doctor had carved the groove behind my glans (what I now know as the sulcus). I wasn't sure what had been done, but I knew it had been an act of cutting. I knew I had been hurt. I learned later that I was missing something.

I was in college when I had my first intact partner; it was then that I discovered what, exactly, was taken from me. When I first saw him without clothes, I was excited to see what a "normal" penis looked like—the way they're supposed to be. What I didn't expect to see is how he got pleasure from things that would've had no effect upon my scarred, diminished penis. Compared to him, I had to go to extremes to get even a little pleasure. I knew I had been robbed—I just hadn't realized the value of what had been taken. This wasn't my first knowledge of the intact penis. I had learned all about it in school and had already developed the intactivist spirit, but this was my first "hands-on" experience of form and function.

In my undergraduate studies in Psychology, I became very close with one of my mentors, now my closest and most trusted friend. Ours was, and still is, a relationship where we're safe to discuss childhood experiences, and feelings of vulnerability, grief, and loss. It was during one of these talks that I brought up my feelings of circumcision. I explained how I was privately grieving my loss and how this violent act was done to me without my consent. I experienced it as a form of rape. She listened closely as I talked about these feelings of powerlessness when I started to go into what I can only call a state of shock. I know that I stopped talking. I remember her asking: "Rick, what are you feeling now?" I went pale and started shaking.

She said she could see the terror in my eyes. "I don't know what's happening," I told her. "I don't have words for this. My hips hurt, like they're being crushed, and my elbows ache, throbbing with my heartbeat, and my groin … it's … burning. Stinging." My heart was racing. I felt dizzy. I wanted to run away, but felt as if I couldn't move. I was re-experiencing some trauma, an old trauma—a memory of something. My circumcision? We were discussing my feelings of loss and powerlessness when this started. We talked about what we had just witnessed and I decided to learn more about it. I was grateful that my friend was with me.

This was back in the early 1990's. My friend and I went to several National Organization of Circumcision Information Resource Centers or NOCIRC[125] events in the Seattle area. During one, we marched to the front door of the company that manufactures the Circumstraint board—the board they use to strap down the newborn.[126] I enjoyed picketing them and being with other intactivists. One of the nurses brought a Circumstraint, which we filled with blood-red carnations.

But when I saw the Circumstraint board, I noticed that its straps cross the long bones mid-thigh and upper arm, not the joints above or below. This design would not put pressure on the hips or the elbows—the places where I had felt pressure in my re-experience. I started to question if those feelings were just my mind filling in what I had imagined had happened to me—my body sympathizing with my interpretation of infant circumcision. I was really confused. It had felt so real. I didn't know what it all meant.

I approached the intactivist nurse who brought the Circumstraint, and asked if there were different designs that maybe strapped at the arms and hips. She explained that the board was not yet used when I was born. It didn't come into use until twelve years after I was born. So I asked her how they restrained the babies when I was born. I'll never forget what she said.

She told me that the nurse stands at the head of the infant and holds the thighs of the child in each hand. She spreads the infant's legs and forces the femurs down pinning the hips to the table and uses her forearms to pin the child's elbows down. This explained exactly what I felt that day! Hips = Pressure, Elbows = Pressure, Penis = Burning pain.

I have no doubt that my body remembers my circumcision that happened on the second day of my life. I relived it that day almost three decades later. I had no way of knowing that it involved my hips and elbows—but that's exactly what came up when I let myself feel the memory that was in my body. I would probably not believe this myself—but I was there. I felt it. And I did not know how I had been held down, so I couldn't have made it up.

---

[125] NOCIRC is an educational non-profit organization based in California. It is committed to securing the birthright of male, female, and intersex children and babies to keep their sex organs intact.

[126] The Circumstraint is a plastic molded board used to immobilize infants for circumcision.

Something in me remembered—remembers. So I know exactly why I'm crying as I write this down.

Rick[127]
52 years
Washington State, USA
3 November 2013

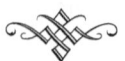

Healing Conversations With Mom

I've resented being circumcised since I was a young child. Once whilst still in primary school, I tried to talk to both my parents but got nowhere. They instantly regurgitated all the crap about it being cleaner and better looking and never having to experience the pain of getting cut as an adult. I backed down. I never told them I disagreed. I never told them I had terribly tight erections. I never told them that I used to wrap my dick in cut up t-shirts to have relief from the constant rubbing and irritation against my underwear.[128]

I decided just over a year ago to talk to my mom about my circumcision. I had in the months prior to talking to her spent a lot of time reading on the topic, including the pros and cons. I read about restoration and explored a foreskin restoration site.

I still stay with my mom and we have a good relationship. She said one night that I had seemed a bit down for a while and asked what was bothering me. Seeing my opportunity to tell her the truth, I told her. The conversation was not as uneasy as I had thought it would be, and for me it has been quite liberating to share my feelings about the one thing that has troubled me for so many years.

Although I told my mom that I did not want her to take on any guilt, a few days later I found her crying. She came and hugged me and told me how sorry she was, and that the day I was circumcised she felt awful. My dad had comforted her, telling her that it was best and it had to be done. I didn't expect this reaction, but it was okay, and I ended up comforting her. This has been one of the biggest moments in my healing, and I have been able to forgive my folks for their poor decision.

Having told her opened up the communication between us on many other things—the girls I'm interested in, what my goals are in life, my beliefs, how my love life is going—all things I never trusted sharing before. This new sharing feels good, healthy. It also was an easy next step to tell her about my planned restoration, so now I don't have to restore in secrecy. In fact, she collected my TLC-X from the post office for me and offered to pay half. A year later, my mom has become something of an intactivist, too, and has spoken to one or two expecting mothers already. She supports me and I truly think that for me telling my mom was the best thing I could have done.

---

[128] By wrapping up his penis, Alfadog was protecting his glans corona from clothing abrasion to avoid painful and irritating stimulation.

My dad, however, is a difficult one. ... I want him to know, but he isn't easy to talk with about anything involving feelings. My folks are recently divorced and he lives nearby. I am writing him a letter. I'm on what must be my twentieth draft attempt to write it in a way that he'll be able to identify where I'm coming from. ... I'll get there.

I think that if you approach the conversation with caring intentions (you're not trying to blame, place guilt or punish), but rather just to share what your experience has been, then I think it can go well, as it has with me. I am so glad that I didn't ignore that feeling of wanting to tell my mom.

Eight months later I haven't mentioned anything to my father. I see him infrequently these days and there hasn't been an opportunity to bring the topic up for discussion. I have always found it difficult to talk to my dad about anything regarding my life. ... I sort of feed him bits I feel comfortable with to stop him from asking! The circumcision topic would be especially awkward with him, and I feel so strongly about it as it was, to my understanding, my dad who decided I had to be circumcised in the first place.

Alfadog
26 years
South Africa
17 January 2012

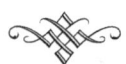

How Being Circumcised At Birth Almost Ruined My Life

Okay, so where should I begin? As the title says, I was circumcised at birth. Luckily, I do not remember it, but sometimes when I think very closely about it I seem to actually be able to very vaguely remember the pain. More like an "intuition" type feeling, but not a memory per se.

It all started when I was around five or six years old. I was baptized and went to Catholic Church when I was a kid. I had a good strong faith in god and that he had the power to help anybody who prayed hard enough and long enough.

One day while I was at daycare I saw some white powder on one of the couches. To this day I'm not sure what it was but I'm pretty sure it was baby powder. I was a strange little kid and when nobody was looking I took a bit and put it in my pants. (Weird, I know, lol.) But, hey, why not? It was always being put on babies. Doing this gave me an erection and it was the first time I noticed my penis. I went to the bathroom and studied it. I noticed it had a scar around it and a dark ring that went from the tip about half way down. I was horrified. I didn't know why it was like that or how it got like that.

Now, I grew up without a father. My mother wasn't ever open about talking to me about sexual organs and stuff so I never (even to this day) felt comfortable saying anything to her. Even at a young age I was embarrassed. So what did I do? For a week straight I went to my bedroom window, pulled out my little penis, and prayed for god to fix me. I prayed so hard and begged and pleaded with god. (Don't worry—We lived in a top floor apartment, so nobody could actually see me doing this, lol). Well, needless to say: nothing ever happened. It completely destroyed all faith I had. But it didn't end there.

Fast forward a few years to middle-school. I still had no knowledge of circumcision or "in-tact" penises. Even though in 5th grade we watched educational videos about puberty, they didn't mention anything about that. I still felt like there was something wrong with me and I lived in constant fear that people might find out. I dreaded and hated thinking about what would happen when I got to high school: I might have to take a shower with other guys in P.E. and they might see me. Oh, just for clarification, I live in the US, so other boys would have been the same. Anyways, in 6th grade and all through middle school I played sports. I loved being active and played baseball and basketball and really enjoyed it, despite being smaller than the other kids and not very good at it. Then, high school ...Luckily we weren't required to take a shower in P.E. This was a huge relief for me. Now some of you might be asking at this point how it was that I got so far in life without visiting a doctor and asking him what might be wrong with it. Well to be completely honest, I didn't have a full physical examination from about age five up to fifteen or sixteen. Crazy, I know.

Anyways, I found out that if I wanted to participate in high school sports, I would need a physical. Sports ended for me. I went to a small school and my graduating class was about thirty people. Everybody played sports—except for me. I never got to build up the jock muscles (or really much muscle at all) and be active other than P.E. because of an inherent fear of the doctor seeing my circumcised penis, which I thought was something incredibly wrong with me.

So basically, there it is. I ended up finding out at around sixteen that I was circumcised and that the darker color and scar were the result of it, and that I was completely normal. Unfortunately, it was too late. I already had the shame and insecurity about my body. I never had a father figure to guide me through it, or happen to see his penis in the shower while growing up, or to ask boy questions.

To this day I feel like something was taken from me. I long so much to have my foreskin and I actively monitor Foregen for ANY sort of progress on a real cure/regeneration of the foreskin. I feel I will never get to experience something important. I am so against circumcision and want to shout to the world (more specifically to the US) how barbaric it is and how they need to leave that sort of decision to the boy for when he grows up.

Boxie7
25 years
Iowa, USA
30 July 2013

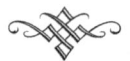

How Circumcision Has Affected My Sex Life

My circumcision as an infant has had many negative permanent changes on me and my sex life.

As a child (six or seven years old) I can remember holding my penis to help protect the sensitive glans from my underwear as I would watch TV.[129] At that time I did not know why, however, I do recall my father saying "Paul, you don't have to hold it. It is not going anywhere."

Unfortunately, as I aged, I was losing sensitivity due to the build up of extra layers of skin coating my unprotected and dried out glans, not to mention all of the nerves that were removed due to my circumcision.

This reduced sensitivity could be one of the reasons it takes me so long to achieve an orgasm. Many mornings and nights my wife would become sore long before I could achieve an orgasm. Although many things cause vaginal soreness, my lack of a natural working foreskin (gliding motion) and reduced sensitivity in my penis certainly didn't help. My wife felt sad (as did I) when I would have to masturbate when I did not reach orgasm during sexual intercourse.

Many factors led to my divorce when I was forty-two, but not being able to enjoy sex with my wife was high on the list. I believe many of my sexual problems (delayed orgasm, lack of sensitivity, and painful erections between the ages of eleven and fifteen) were the result of my circumcision and lack of a complete (intact) natural functioning foreskin and penis.

I never knew how much sensation I had lost until I started restoring my foreskin. However, attempting to re-grow a protective skin covering for my glans has been one of the most challenging things I have ever attempted in my life (including a four year college degree). I must work so hard to try to re-grow (as much as possible) what I already had but which was taken from me without my consent.

---

[129] Paul is here referring to the annoying rather than pleasurable sensations detected by the protopathic nerve endings in most of the glans surface. (Henry Head, *Studies in Neurology*, Vol. 1 (London: Hodder & Stoughton, 1920), 277.)

After partially restoring my foreskin, my ex-wife and I are back living together and trying to work things out.

Paul
52 years
Florida, USA
25 October 2013

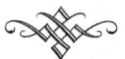

Inadequate

My circumcision is something that I did not really think critically about until I was around nineteen or twenty years old, and I've grown more frustrated and aggrieved about it since then. Now I'm consumed with regret for what was done to me; I hate it so much. While I have emotional and psychological problems that prevent me from having relationships and sex, I don't think I can bear having sex while feeling this way about how I am physically.

Even though I hadn't reflected all that much on my circumcised state until my late teens, I've always felt like something was wrong with my penis. I remember noticing problems with my glans and how dry and cracked it was. I remember thinking that it might be because I wasn't cleaning enough or something.

Another issue I had was that I have hair growing on my shaft, covering between a third and a half of my penis, and I was very self-conscious about that, both from the looks and the physical discomfort of it. I've since then realized that the skin that most of my shaft hair grows on is probably scrotal skin, i.e. skin pulled up from my scrotum, since it's so different from both the inner foreskin left and the outer shaft skin. It's thicker, a different color, and it has bumps on it (like found on my scrotum.) Take that and the fact that my skin is pretty tight when I'm erect, I think I probably had a more severe cut than most.

I'm having such a difficult time dealing with every single flaw. I feel completely mutilated and inadequate, and I don't know how I'll ever learn to cope with this as a sexual person. Often I wish I didn't even have any sexual feelings, because every time it just reminds me of how fucked up I am. I fear the very real possibility that there may not be a recourse for me, that I may just be some sexual cripple my entire life. I constantly fantasize about not having been circumcised, trying to imagine what I'd look and feel like if I was intact. That obviously doesn't help things.

For me, I don't really blame my parents or anything, I feel like they were victims of cultural indoctrination like I was. I've talked to my mother about it a little bit before, and I asked her why they had it done. She basically said that it was just what was always done and that it was more of a question of why not, rather than why, which is obviously stupid reasoning. I didn't push the issue because I didn't want to make her feel bad, and I didn't want to have to reveal too many personal feelings.

I'm thinking about talking to my dad about it, but I don't know if I should. I really don't know what to expect from him (it could go either way for all I know) and I don't know if I'd get anything out of it. The bottom line is, even if it went as well as possible, it's not going to undo any of the damage that has been done to me.

Mark
25 years
California, USA
October - November 2011

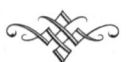

Is My Sexual Dysfunction Due To Circumcision?

The story of my circumcision is like that of many other men born in the late eighties. Both of my parents are atheists or at least agnostic. They made it no secret that they had me circumcised as a baby at the doctor's recommendation. We don't talk openly about sexual topics, but they explained what it was and why they had it done and it never really bothered me. My father is circumcised and, as far as I know, his father was, too. I'm not sure about my mother's side of the family, but she's fairly certain that her brothers are.

Now here is where my story differs from the myriad of angry and tragic ones I've read. I discovered masturbation at age twelve and I now realize that circumcision caused some difficulties. For example, I never understood why using my hand felt better than humping and simulating sex. I was Coverage Index Two (CI-2)[130] and I actually thought that bumping my skin up against the corona was the wrong way to masturbate, but it was still my preferred method. But despite this, masturbation felt fantastic. In fact, around age fifteen or sixteen I remember having extremely powerful orgasms that made my body spasm and sometimes left me with a "floating on air" feeling. They also gave me a great night's sleep and on more than one occasion I woke up next to a puddle of drool.

However, by my early twenties I noticed that these orgasms were becoming less and less frequent. Additionally I felt less during masturbation and it took longer to reach a climax. I've also noticed that my libido has dropped. I still have a sex drive, but whereas in the past my imagination was enough to give me throbbing erections, now it only gets me to "half mast" most of the time. The only theory I have right now is that the high levels of testosterone partially compensated for my missing and damaged tissue. Also, I grew up in the Internet age, so if I had a hard time getting excited, pornography was always just a few clicks away.

I thought my problems had something to do with aging or that I had injured myself. (I've never used prone masturbation or any other odd techniques.) But, one day when trying to get myself excited, I looked at a pornographic video online and saw that the man had his foreskin. I did a bit of research and had the usual shocked reaction that my sexual dysfunction was due at

---

[130] The Coverage Index is a classification system that gives numerical values to describe the length of foreskin; CI-1 means no foreskin (i.e. all has been removed by circumcision) and CI-10 means there is enough foreskin to overhang the top of the glans. See http://www.newforeskin.biz/.

least in part (if not entirely) to my circumcision.

It didn't take me long to decide to pursue restoration and I have been using exclusively manual methods 1 and 2[131] for the last year about one to two hours a day over multiple sessions. I like the progress I've made so far but I'm currently in the CI-3 "ugly duckling" stage.

I realize this should make me optimistic, but I actually have a pretty hard time with it sometimes. I know I can have satisfying sexual experiences but it's been years and sometimes it feels like they're gone for good. I know people are concerned about putting things on a numerical scale and talking about "whole body orgasms," but I'm more interested in slow rhythmic intercourse. What I'm really hoping for is to enjoy the act of sex itself, not just the "big finish."

Zoop
24 years old
Ohio, USA
November 2013

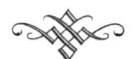

---

[131] "Manual Tugging: Method 1,"
http://www.restoringforeskin.org/blog/2009/05/manual-tugging-method-1 (accessed 3 February 2014).

It Starts With A Piece

Circumcision for me has been a whirl of mixed emotions. Overall, I can assure you that none of them are good. When I think about my circumcision, I have to face a hard fact: I have been altered, and in a very personal way. I am reminded that as a baby boy, being born as I was, I was just not good enough.

Most people I have encountered don't tend to think circumcision can cut so deeply, but in fact, it is a very deep cut. I find people left and right circumcising their children with no qualms, thinking they're doing the best for their child. To justify themselves they'll say, "It's just a piece of skin." And, thus, with such reasoning, they circumcise their children: They cut away a piece. However, from my experience, the effects of circumcision create much more. Ultimately, the results of being circumcised create a mosaic, because it is not one piece, but thousands of pieces building up. This mosaic created out of me and many other men is in all essence something ugly—something which should not have been made. Simply and graphically put, a mosaic is formed of blood and flesh, of torture and screams, of pain and psychosis.

A lot of circumcised men are aware of their very personal unchosen alterations. But, as men we are taught to not express our emotions: it is rare you will hear a man express how he feels, especially if he is bothered by his circumcision. As men, one of our utmost inner values is to build up security and confidence in ourselves. Yet where can one have confidence if he knows he wasn't good enough from birth, that he had to be altered? It is no secret that as men we constantly obsess over our sexual prowess, and try our best to maintain our sexual securities. Among many more manhood worries, we worry if our penises are big enough to do the job right, if they'll bring our partners the best pleasure they can have, if they'll bring ourselves the best pleasure we can have, if they'll impress another person.

When it all comes down to it, circumcision is the removal of a piece. It all starts with a piece, a piece of skin. With the cutting of the skin comes a piece of blood. With a piece of blood comes a piece of pain. With a piece of pain come the pieces of screams for help. With no answer to the cry for help comes a piece of helplessness. With helplessness, this pain becomes a torture. With torture, the state of the mind is altered, and, in the end, a piece of the soul is taken.

But sadly, the actions are long lasting, taking in time more pieces. As I have matured, I've discovered from not having my foreskin that there is a piece of my sexuality I will never know or discover, so another piece is gone. As I research circumcision, I learn there are tens of thousands of nerve endings with which I will never feel, creating a sense of a loss of sexual fortitude, so there goes a piece of my strength. I read that these nerve endings bring the most pleasure to a man, so I have learned a piece of my pleasure is gone. I read on, and learn that the foreskin helps protect the head of the penis from sensitivity loss and from becoming dirty. Here three pieces are now gone: a piece of my cleanliness, a piece of my sensitivity, and most importantly, a piece of my security.

With this knowledge, I become angry as I recognize this surgery on me was done without my permission. Sadly, it was done when I could never have given permission even if I had wanted to, for I could not speak. No child comes out of the womb knowing to communicate with words, so a piece of my voice was taken. This causes more than just anger, for there's more than one piece of my emotions: There's a piece for sadness at the loss, a piece for confusion as to why, a piece for jealousy as I learn of luckier men who have the choice to remain whole.

As I age, I learn my sensitivity decreases greatly and I have much difficulty utilizing my penis. I can barely bring myself pleasure, let alone my partner pleasure, so there goes a piece of my confidence. In light of these sexual difficulties and with the intention to salvage my abilities, I resort to pharmaceuticals for aid for erectile dysfunction, so there goes a piece of my joy in bringing pleasure to my lover. There also goes a piece of my success in the self-fulfillment of the acquisition of my own pleasure.

After these frustrations I cast aside my manhood, my penis, leaving it still a part of my body, but of no use to me other than to expel waste. So, another piece of me withers away: my masculinity, the piece that signified me as a man in the first place, that told the people of the world, "I am a man," at my birth.

On top of what was taken away from the cut itself, the reasons for circumcision also take away many pieces from us. The reason "one has a lower STD acquisition rate if circumcised" takes away a piece of my trustworthiness. They assume I will not take precautionary measures to have safe sex, even though it is clear a condom is cheaper, more effective, and more reasonable than making a permanent cut to my penis. The reason "it's cleaner" takes a piece of my intelligence, assuming that I am not smart enough to maintain my personal hygiene. The reasons "it's tradition" and of

"I want him to look like daddy" or "I want my son to look like me" takes a piece of individuality, for no two men are ever the same.

Ultimately, being circumcised without consent has taken a piece of my freedom, by my not having the choice of who I want to be.[132]

Over my lifetime my mosaic is slowly building. When all the pieces are placed together, the mosaic shows only a tragic scene of a victim, of an inner demon, a man-made creation gone awry, an atrocity. After all, it all starts with one piece. What is not realized, I think, is of all the pieces taken in circumcision, what stands out is that the most important pieces of a man himself are removed. All of the pieces are those which we attribute most to being a man: freedom, individuality, security, success, joy, trustworthiness, having a voice, intelligence, strength, confidence, and masculinity.

Now, upon the personal reflection of my circumcision, assuredly I have felt the pain and heartache of the pieces of my self and soul being damaged. Yet, as a man, I still hold onto my virtues. As a man, I take pride in never giving up, and in exerting dedication to being the man who betters himself. Though my circumcision has slighted me, I resort not to bitterness, though I have experienced it.

In my discoveries of life so far, I have learned I can restore my foreskin. Sure, it sounds downright silly as a proposition. Ultimately I wish I never had been cut in the first place so that I would never have to endure this. But being a circumcised man, the restoration of my foreskin is my one saving grace to self-healing, to self-preservation, to not giving in to the bitterness of being damaged. I am instead turning my vision toward being hopeful.

Although I can never fully undo all the damage to my penis and the pieces of myself which were damaged as a result, I do have one choice. I can try my best to rebuild myself and, in my self-awareness, I can also reach out to others to let them know about circumcision. I can help them make informed decisions, so that the future men of this world will not suffer as I and many others have through our unfortunate deprivation of never having had the chance or choice to a whole and complete body.

---

[132] This is the Open Future Principle, proposed by legal philosopher Joel Feinberg. See J. Feinberg, "The child's right to an open future," in *Freedom and Fulfillment: Philosophical Essays* (Princeton, Princeton University Press, 1992).

And in this case, finally, it starts with a piece: a piece of hope, a piece of knowledge, a piece of inspiration, a piece of altruism, and a piece of love. Ultimately, building piece upon piece creates a mosaic, this time of the celebration of life.

Kohiro Hakuya
26 years
Japan
14 June 2012

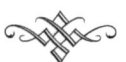

Living With A Botched Circumcision

I was born in the military hospital at Fort Stewart, Georgia. My parents were devout Christians who also gave in to all of the hypocrisy regarding male versus female genital mutilation. I was circumcised, and my grandma told me that I held my father's hand while he let the doctors rip open the foreskin of my penis and crush away the 'excess skin' containing thousands upon thousands of nerve endings. Little did those quack military doctors know, they left an incision on the bottom of the circumcision line (underside of the penis), which eventually ripped completely open in later years.

I do not remember exactly how old I was, but I remember the pain very vividly. When I was around three or four, I was sitting in the bathtub while playing with my Power Rangers action figures. I situated my legs in a crisscross applesauce position (aka tailor sitting) because that's how I was taught to sit. I felt an excruciating ripping sensation starting from the tip of my penis. It continued to happen for approximately one hour while in the bathtub, and blood was surrounding my naked body.

Paranoia was setting in, and I did not want my parents to know. What I did was wait until the ripping sensation stopped, then drained the bloody water and put my underwear on. By the time I stepped out of the bath, I quit bleeding and there was just raw, exposed meat. I saw that the skin of my penis was completely separated.

I did not tell my parents, because I was afraid that they might blame me for masturbating or they might tell the doctor to cut off more nerve endings by trying to fix the current situation. I just let the huge rip heal over a period of seven months, ignoring the intense pain it caused me.

I was also afraid of telling my parents of anything sexual because they were Christian.[133] Sex is a no-no. You don't talk about sex when you are THAT age! I lived in a Christian home and was forced to go to Church whenever they felt like it, and I was pretty much sheltered my whole life. Being a "military brat" as well as an only child, I lived a very secluded and repressed lifestyle. My dad going off to fight in whatever wars they had at the time for more than three times didn't help the situation(s) either.

Long story short with my parents, they got rid of me as a teenager and I lived with my grandma for approximately two years before I headed off to college after my eighteenth birthday. I did not like finding out that my intact father

---

[133]For a comprehensive account of how religion interferes with normal sexual psychology see Darrel Ray, *Sex and God* (Kansas: IPC Press, 2012).

allowed my penis to be partially castrated without my consent. I was abused mentally (somewhat physically) with Christianity (mostly maternally) and my dad listened to everything she said and ran with it.

My current situation is that I am stuck with fucked up genitalia for the rest of my human existence on this planet. I will never experience a full body orgasm with my penis due to the fact that along with the male G-spot and nerve rich foreskin being amputated, I have had the entire bottom of my genitals ripped open from the doctors leaving a rip in the scar line.

I started restoring around 2011, but I have had minimal results with taping methods. I came out publicly as an intactivist during the latter half of 2012 and will remain one until the day I die. I want to sue, but considering I was circumcised in a military hospital in Georgia, I don't think that will be possible. I am a poor college student and I don't know how that would work out.

I created a video when I was seventeen exposing the harm of what neonatal male circumcision does to a child. YouTube censored my video and removed it from their database. I had to re-upload the video. Too many individuals do not talk about how circumcision has negatively impacted their lives, and that is also one of the reasons why it persists in the United States.

Vance
18 years
Oklahoma, USA
17 September 2013

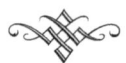

Masturbation Cure

I was born in Brussels, Belgium, in September 1930. Catholicism is the state religion of Belgium, meaning that essentially no one attends church anymore. Of my large extended family, only my maternal grandmother was a practicing Catholic. At that time, medical articles reported that circumcision cured masturbation, and that masturbation is the cause of blindness and of mental retardation. Mental illnesses were hidden as much as possible, and never mentioned. A family with a known case of mental retardation had difficulty finding a suitable spouse for its young adults. I remember my maternal grandmother frequently whispering the name of a family cursed with a retarded relative.

Probably in early 1935, my maternal grandmother took me to an old doctor and whispered to him. Without examining me, the doctor told me to stop playing by myself. He must have meant to play with myself, which in French is expressed with the same words. Although my sister was still in diapers and in a playpen, I had been raised to never question an adult. Truly, no matter how hard I try, I do not remember having done anything that my parents had forbidden, but so many events from that age are lost to my memory.

Sometime later, my grandmother took me to a hospital, where I was put to sleep with chloroform, a sweet, nauseating smell. After waking up, and told by a nun to eat a custard, I threw up. The nun called me a dirty sinner (*pécheur* in French). I do not recall physical pain from the procedure, only something vague, when I had to urinate.

Some time later, I asked my mother why was I a dirty fisherman.[134] (I had never heard the word *pécheur*.) My mother became very upset, and asked who called me that. I just said the nun at the hospital. My mother told me never to talk about it, and I did not, until I asked my father, in 1953. My father was born in Brooklyn, New York, but got his MBA in Belgium, where he met and married my mother.

In 1953, living with my father while waiting for my mother and sister to join us in the U.S., I asked why he had let me be circumcised. My father had always planned to bring us to the U.S., but my mother kept postponing the decision, not ready to leave her parents or the way of life she was accustomed to. Knowing that practically all boys in the U.S. were circumcised, like he had been, my father thought that it would be easier for me to assimilate, and actually, he was right. While enrolled at Brooklyn Polytechnic, the swimming for P.E. was at the local YMCA, where nude

---

[134] The French word for fisherman is *pêcheur*.

swimming was the norm. Seeing that the majority of the students were circumcised, I did feel more "American."

Going back in time, my mother postponing our moving to the U.S. forced us to spend World War II under German occupation. I believe on the last Wednesday of June 1944, soon after D-day, German officers, soldiers and their dogs came to the school. One by one, we had to go in a small room and drop our pants in front of an officer. The officer laughed, pointing at my crotch, and said something (in German) to the soldiers, who had guns and dogs on a leash. He then told me to put my pants back on, and again spoke in German to the soldiers. One of the soldiers said something to his dog, and the dog barked and leaped toward me, but did not touch me since the leash was too short. The soldier took me by the shoulder and led me outside through the backdoor, then in the back of a truck.

There were two much younger, crying boys on the bench along the left side of the truck, and two soldiers, each with a dog on the opposite side. I was pushed to sit next to the boys, and the soldier who took me sat in front of me. He started to laugh and talk in German. His dog again growled and jumped toward me, and the other two soldiers started to laugh and have the dogs jump and growl at the other boys. Soon, the truck driver came to close the tarpaulin, and the truck drove off. The soldiers kept laughing and teasing us with the dogs. After what felt like a long time, the truck stopped and we were taken into a large building, which I think is the Solvay Institute.[135] (Later on, I learned that German scientists were conducting research on the effects of beta radiation.)

We were taken to a hallway next to a large laboratory, in which I saw a large machine with a running belt and several men in white lab coats. (When I was at Brooklyn Polytech, there was a Van de Graaf generator, which I immediately recognized; the physics instructor explained to me that it had been used to generate high voltages to simulate beta radiation, which of course is made of electrons. I am not sure that the soldiers took me to the Solvay Research Institute. The name was mentioned by the physics teaching assistant when I said that I had seen a Van de Graaf machine in Belgium.)

In the hallway, a Belgian man (he spoke French without an accent) told us to take our clothes off. When I took my shirt off, the man smiled and said that I was lucky to be a sinner instead of a Jew. (At the beginning of the German occupation, after a medical visit, I was given a round dog tag to show that I was a sinner, and not a Jew; the other boys had their tag in the shape of a cross, except the Jews, who had a Star of David tag.) The man also told me

---

[135] A Belgian chemical company founded in 1863.

that I was too big for the box, and that only two boys were needed that day. He then talked in German to the soldiers, then gave me back my clothes, and said it was my lucky day.

The three soldiers then took me back to the school in the same truck and still had fun scaring me with the dogs. The trucks and soldiers who were there earlier had all left. One of the soldiers who had brought one of the boys then took my hand and brought me to the school principal. This soldier did not tell his dog to bark at me, and kept my hand while we walked through the school hallways. Although I was too scared to think clearly, later on I realized that some soldiers were reluctantly doing their jobs.

After the soldier left, the principal told me that I was lucky, but that a second time, I would not be, and thus I was not supposed to say a word about what had happened, especially not to the other students, nor even to my parents. Although at the time I assumed that principal was responsible for the German soldiers coming to the school, about ten years ago I was told that he probably had not given the name of any Jewish student, and that was the reason for the inspection. The principal gave me a sealed envelope to bring to my teacher. The teacher opened it, and looked at me in a strange way, but simply told me to sit at my desk. The whole ordeal had only taken little more than two hours, yet it seemed like a whole day. I am not sure that I could have kept silent about it, because I was still terrified when I came home that afternoon.

About an hour later, we had an air raid alert. American B-17s were bombing railways, bridges, and convoys almost daily, and English planes were bombing at night. As usual, we went to the cellar, but this time, bombs had fallen so close that almost as soon as the ground shook, plaster dust got in the cellar. To keep from suffocating, we were used to having wet pieces of old clothes in the cellar, and we covered our faces. Coming out of the cellar, most of the windows were broken. One bomb had fallen in front of the house and a series of them had destroyed the house on the other side of the back yard, and then, across the back street, a whole coliseum used by stationed German soldiers. If it had not been for the coincidence of the bombing on the same day, I could not have kept silent in front of my parents.

The first person I told was my wife, only a few days after we were married in 1957. It was very emotional to talk about it, and my wife's understanding and caring then is probably responsible for our happy marriage. I have told my children and grandchildren, and lately have shared these memories with men I meet at the National Organization of Restoring Men (NORM) meetings. I do not get as emotional anymore. However, I am still terrified of big dogs, and I know that dogs feel it, because they always snarl, bark, or run after me.

On a completely different level, the doctor who circumcised me took too much skin on the left, causing strongly leftward bending erections. This could have made our wedding night into a disaster. But my wife was patient, understanding, and somewhat of a gymnast. She also suggested I wear my penis to the right in tight briefs. Although very uncomfortable at first, it did help a lot. I only wish I had been smart enough at the time to realize that with continuous stretching, I could have restored my foreskin. After I found that non-surgical foreskin restoration was possible, my wife approved of it, but unfortunately, after a very long illness, she passed away in 2010. I still keep on restoring, knowing that she would have encouraged me to do it.

Alfred
83 years
Texas, USA
26 October 2013

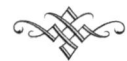

Alfred died on 11 March 2014.

When asked to contribute to this book, Alfred responded "It is an honor that you would consider my reminiscences about having been circumcised."

"Alfred had a warm heart, and a strength of character that inspired many. I miss Alfred's indomitable spirit, and I often think of him, as one does those we love." – Roy

Men Do Indeed Complain

My earliest recollections about circumcision include me at about eleven years old asking my mom what circumcision meant. She explained that they take some nasty extra skin from the penis and guys are much better off as a result. She said I should be glad it was done to me. (It would be thirty more years before I learned my father was never circumcised.)

In my twenties I started hearing things that made me realize Mom was wrong; that circumcision wasn't strictly good; that most of the world's men were happily intact. But it wasn't until I heard Dr Jim Bigelow interviewed on the radio about his book *The Joy of Uncircumcising*[136] in 1995 that I really understood how even a well performed circumcision affected sex negatively.

When I was thirty-three, I realized intellectually that I was missing something good and I was getting a little pissed off about it. But the restoration methods Bigelow was touting involved tapes and weights, and I just couldn't see myself heading down that road. Even if foreskin was the greatest thing since unsliced bread, I wasn't convinced that restoring would deliver a great enough degree of a rejuvenation to warrant the hassles that I imagined taping involved. Sex with my wife was fine. I just assumed up to this point that my ability to last a very long time in bed was due to my diligent efforts to be the best possible lover.

By age thirty-eight my attitude had shifted. In ten years of happy marriage my wife had never succeeded at finishing me orally despite sincere and concerted effort. And by this point I could literally go all night at intercourse with her and then only experience orgasm if I really concentrated and she talked dirty and stuff. A few times we gave up on my orgasm after numerous orgasms for her. She'd say she was getting rubbed raw. We would need a few days off before trying again.

Was my lack of sensation just due to aging? Surely that was possible, but I knew my dad—single and sixty-four years old—was having quite a busy dating life. Maybe my vasectomy a few years earlier had something to do with it? No, I was fine for quite a while after that snip. Why is nothing else about me aging so badly? I tried slathering copious quantities of lotion on my penis every day for a month, but at my next medical check-up my doctor noticed an infected follicle. I told him what I was up to and about my desire to get more supple and sensitive. He said: "Better stick with tough and

---

[136] Jim Bigelow, *The Joy of Uncircumcising!: Exploring Circumcision: History, Myths, Psychology, Restoration, Sexual Pleasure and Human Rights* (Aptos: Hourglass Publishing, 1992).

leathery." Thanks, Doc.

I thought again of restoring and went online to learn the latest. At the time there were some new tapeless methods that seemed to make non-surgical foreskin restoration less of a hassle, but ready-made devices were expensive and the home-made devices baffled me. I found an Australian's write-up of the pill tube (film canister) tape method. I figured I could try the tapes for a few months and if it really seemed to be producing desirable changes, I would then invest in a tapeless device.

On 1 April 2001, I told my wife I planned on stuffing my glans into a short tube, rolling shaft skin forward around the tube, and taping it in place against the tube. She started to say "That's ridiculous! You got me, April Fool." But I told her I needed her support, not ridicule. I would wear a tension strap pretty much 24/7, and she would need to warn me when it was a good time to have my penis available for recreation. After I showed her the pile of articles I had printed out from the Internet, I got her full encouragement.

I made great quick restoration progress. The method I chose allowed me to keep my glans bathed in lotion 24/7, so I got noticeably more supple and sensitive within a few weeks. I was so struck by the improvement I wanted to start telling people. I spent hours every night online advising other men about how and why they could restore.

I even wrote a letter to my employer's director of human resources. I didn't tell him about my own restoring project, but I explained how circumcision is destructive and suggested the company should save money by renegotiating our health plan to exclude coverage for routine circumcision. I wasn't merely meddling in his duties since my job title was "cost savings engineer." He went into a rage with my boss and I was fired a few months later when the company made 9/11 related cutbacks. Before I was fired, I had started to dabble in tapeless methods. I even ordered an expensive device, but the maker was temporarily out of business due to a relocation, and I got a PayPal refund. Once my eight months of unemployment was underway, I had plenty of time to research and refine tapeless restoring devices. When I accepted my next engineering job, I didn't tell them I had a little sideline making foreskin restoration devices and selling them on eBay.

My devices got popular, and in 2004 I incorporated as a foreskin restoration business, while still working nine to five as an engineer. I would spend my lunch hour trimming devices and packing orders. Over the next four years as the business grew I had to get better and better about exploiting every free minute so I could keep up with device demand, be a good dad, and also put in eight honest hours at my day job. For example I would leave the house with my shoes untied and tend to that at the first traffic light rather than spend an extra minute at home. I would prepare sub-assemblies with one hand while driving sixty miles per hour down the highway. Every minute saved meant an extra minute of sleep.

One time a day-job colleague—call him Angelo—asked me to discuss a project over lunch. Since Angelo's family was from Mexico I guessed that he might not be circumcised and I decided to confide in him why I had no time at lunch for his meeting. I told him how I was moonlighting and needed lunch time to get out today's orders. Of the few people at my day job who knew about my sideline, Angelo was perhaps the wrong one to tell, since shortly after that he became my boss.

I assumed that at some point every man who was as odd as me and willing to tug himself a new foreskin would eventually find me, and the demand would then dry up. In a shocking development, the demand for foreskin restoration devices just kept growing by about twenty percent per year. By 2008 to keep up with orders I was getting four hours of sleep per weeknight if I was lucky. My efficiency at work was probably suffering but Angelo was a compassionate boss. He would occasionally privately ask if I felt my sideline was allowing me to give one hundred percent to my day job. By April of 2008 I finally answered honestly, only because I had done the math and decided my family could live on what the foreskin restoration devices earned us, as long as we made some cutbacks in consumption and my wife continued to work as a CPA twenty hours per week. So we phased me out of my day job by June. We didn't anticipate my wife's employer closing that same month, or the economy abruptly tanking.

Howard Stern saved us. I had been lucky to get some positive publicity over the years, including appearing in a BBC documentary and being interviewed by major newspapers and *Time* magazine. If those things had come to the attention of my day job employer, I felt I could explain myself and perhaps stay employed. But it was only after quitting my day job that I could fearlessly answer the call when Howard Stern announced in August 2008 that he was having a pretty penis contest.

I volunteered for Howard's contest, paid my own way to New York, and showed up at Howard's radio/TV studio secretly wearing a foreskin restoration device under my clothes. When it was my turn to drop my trunks and reveal my penis to the celebrity judge (*Star Trek*'s George Takei), there I was with full restoring apparatus on display.

Howard and his crew expressed a sincere interest in the what and the how and the why of restoring, and Howard put a restoration web link on his hugely trafficked web site alongside the summary of that day's show events. I didn't win the penis contest but device sales volume for 2008 stayed level with 2007, which in hindsight could have been a lot worse given the magnitude of the global recession.

Subsequent years saw the twenty percent annual demand growth pattern re-established. I continue to innovate and improve quality and efficiency, and the restoration device market also continues to broaden and welcome new players. So, it looks like we'll be able to continue to make a living in a way that makes us the luckiest family alive. It's truly a dream to have a calling that leaves the world a better place and touches people in such a personal way.

But every week I get letters from men that break my heart. Some men are looking for help to undo artifacts of infant circumcision that are just horrid. Having never compared penises with other men, they don't know just how sub-par their hack job is and I get the job of breaking it to them.

Other men come to me in anguish having recently elected to get cut as adults. The email contact might start with questions about how to treat tight foreskin (phimosis). I explain the simple stretching techniques and the next reply says: "I KNEW it. Damn! Why did I let that quack cut off the best part of my penis?"

Some of the worst circumcision effects we see have nothing to do with the competence of a surgeon. Skin bridges, where the surviving shaft skin adheres to the freshly gouged glans during healing, are quite common. The fault for these lies with the caregiver who is a layperson, likely unaware of what normal healing is supposed to look like. But that doesn't excuse the cutter at all. It was unnecessary surgery and inadequate consultation regardless of how skillfully the cutting tools were wielded. Skin bridges pose a special challenge for restoration device users. I'm happy to do the custom fitting for these cases at no extra charge.

But even a "perfect" circumcision alters sex dramatically. Foreskin amputation removes the sleeve of mobile skin that would protect the suppleness and sensitivity of the glans. It eliminates the possibility of the frictionless gliding mode of stimulation. It excises thousands of pleasure receptive nerve endings on a surface which has the same area as a 3" x 5" index card.[137] That's a lot of sexual interface destroyed, usually without its owner's consent. That's why men continue to find me, over a dozen per day.

---

[137]A 3 inch x 5 inch (7.6 cm x 12.7 cm) index card is the equivalent total area of both surfaces of a typical foreskin.

I've helped over 20,000 men since I started making foreskin restoration devices and, sadly, there is no end in sight.

Ron
51 years
Illinois, USA
13 December 2013

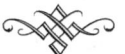

Message To My Parents

I am writing this because I wanted to try and explain things to you. I am concerned that if I try and do it face-to-face or on the phone, I will either clam up or it will just come out garbled and I don't think that will help in the circumstances. You will obviously have noticed that I have not been as communicative recently as previously and I want to explain. Whether you want to hear and what happens from here on in is up to you.

I am not in a good place at the moment. This, along with so many other aspects of things that have happened in my life, I would have to put firmly onto the fact that you both decided it was acceptable to mutilate me, (presumably as an eight day old baby). This was based, presumably just on some "religion" that dictates that this kind of action is necessary, appropriate, and suitable for any parent to visit on their defenseless, unconsenting child.

The amount of grief and upset that this single action has caused me throughout my life is incalculable. I felt "different" to my peers as a small child and then tried to cut myself down there on two occasions to try and make things look more "normal." I felt inadequate as a teenager and adult because a key part of my body has been removed without my consent. I feel as an adult I have been violated and have been sentenced to a second-rate substandard sex life and now am suffering problems due to lack of sensitivity and sensation caused by years of chafing on parts of my body which should not be exposed to the elements. These—and much more besides—have got me to this situation that I'm now in.

Please do not try to delude anyone that a "little piece of skin" was removed and shouldn't have caused any problems. I have done LOTS of research over the years and have a full appreciation of just what has been done to me. It left me with a lifetime of issues and also causing problems for any partners in my life: causing friction problems, chafing, you name it…

What I cannot get my head around is WHY. Whether or not this is part of a religious doctrine is neither here nor there—did it never cross your mind to not go through with that particular act and just carry on with the rest of the religion? At least it may have meant that it would not have completely turned me against the religion, ensuring that I'd never have anything further to do with it in my life or my children's lives. Surely, even if you have had to endure being mutilated in the name of the religion, did it never cross your mind that this is and was wholly unnecessary? People say that the Internet was obviously not available in the past, so people "didn't know about" this or that, but even so, SURELY it must have crossed your mind that people have evolved over millions of years and, therefore, the skin is there for a reason?

I simply cannot get my head around this—I do not understand how this can equate to the first role of any parent to their child: that of care and instilling trust with that child. As soon as the parent lets that child be mutilated—simply for dogma—that trust is broken as irreparably as the child's genital integrity.

So, that is why I am feeling awkward and uncomfortable with you both at the moment. Please be assured this is not some flash in the pan thing that I have suddenly discovered on the Internet or that I am having some sort of psychotic episode: This has been a real issue in my life since I was old enough to determine that I didn't look the same as my friends at school. Whether or not my brothers feel the same, I honestly couldn't say. Maybe you need to have a conversation with them if you feel able.

I don't want to lose touch with you both—notwithstanding anything else, it's not fair to my daughters—they've lost enough recently without my adding further to that. However, I don't feel I can bottle things up any more. I am now taking steps to try and restore some of what I have lost—yes, it is possible to do that by inducing mitosis over five or more years—and have been doing so for the last six months. I guess I don't expect you to understand, but then clearly you never did in the first place or I would not be needing to sit here writing this message to you.

Alan
45 years
United Kingdom
12 December 2013

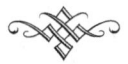

My Experience Of Two Circumcising Cultures

Complaining about being circumcised is like complaining about having to shave each morning. Being born in Iran, a child's birth consists of stage one: in which parents are in awe of the beautiful child that just came to life, and if that child was a male all their attention directly goes, "How I can get this boy circumcised the best way possible?"

I was born into a fairly agnostic family. My mother and the rest of her family were really close and I was often with an aunt, my mother's uncles or aunts, or some relative that we were close to. My father was the only man in his family that did not keep faith, and although he was not necessarily the black sheep, he was never as close to members of his family besides his mother and grandmother, as Mom was to hers.

With that said, my circumcision was not done due directly to the Islamic tradition of *Khitan* or in Persian *Khatne*. Rather, since Iran is politically Muslim (funny enough most citizens in this day and age are non-religious there), it is the same tradition as here in America. Here too, it is also seen as clean and tidy.

I was a month old when I was cut. I went with my mother and grandmother to the hospital to get cut. From what I've been told I had a special machine to give me an even cut, and the doctor said that they gave me what was known as a "half-circumcision." My mom becomes teary eyed each time she remembers it, only describing it as there being so much blood. If anything, I feel worse for my mother than myself for having to see me go through that.

But I still ask myself, if in those four weeks after I was born, had it not occurred to my parents even once that they didn't need to cut me? I'm sure they did it out of love and to care for me, and thinking about it now of course I say, "Damn, what would have happened if they decided not to cut me? Would I still be the same man?" Of course, their choosing to circumcise me did not in the least bit change my views on them. If anything, I love them more for trying to care for me.

At the age of three I moved to California, and felt right at home a couple weeks after I arrived. My guess is at the age of four I saw my first uncircumcised penis. I remember it really clearly: three boys and I were peeing in a urinal all at the same time from different angles. I'm assuming the one on the left was cut but the other penis looked weird. When I asked my mom about it she said that "Americans have it like that, but it's more clean to not have it." I had no idea "that" meant my skin was cut; I just thought they hid the tip in while my mom took the tip of my penis out of my shaft. For the longest time I remember trying to tuck my glans inside my shaft so I can have my penis like that (likely so I could show it off to my friends at pre-school).

Growing up, I began masturbating at the age of fourteen. Truth be told, it wasn't all that great, but it did release some of the sexual tension teenage boys have when testosterone levels skyrocket. I thought that the amazing experience people talked about was the difference between sex and masturbation. I couldn't help but want more then, because something just didn't click that I felt was supposed to.

The whole circumcision aspect never got to me. I would just always like to say that Americans had it lucky for not being circumcised, but in all actuality, almost everyone I knew was cut. In locker rooms seeing that one uncircumcised penis (usually from an East Asian or Latin American) was always an unexpected shock.

Life went normally until the day came when I found about the harms of circumcision. Our friends were out shooting a film for a small advertising campaign when someone said, "Some chick thinks uncircumcised cocks are gross." At this, funny enough, a Hispanic friend of mine rolled his eyes cursing for realizing there was another reason he would never get it on with that girl. Immediately another friend of mine said in retaliation that the foreskin has half the nerves of the penis.

Now I want to ask you a question: When you hear awful news and are in a group of people, how awful is that feeling when your throat clenches and you need to act normal? When the seconds turn into minutes and the minutes into hours? All I wanted to do was go home and look this up, hoping he was wrong.

Before I continue, I think it's important to address that growing up I was a very competitive person. As an idol of mine said, "I can accept failure, everyone fails at something. But I can't accept not trying." Each time I wanted to improve or gain something I would work to get it, even if it meant hours in the gym or in the library. I always wanted to win and learn how to get better, but here I realized I couldn't do a thing to get back one of my most vital organs, something that I never consented to being taken from me. I couldn't accept it. I thought to myself, "Even if I grew my foreskin, would it ever be the same?" I pray that Foregen[138] will work someday and bless my life. Soon enough I was in a state of denial trying to tell myself that foreskin

---

[138] Foregen is an organization that hopes to eventually provide circumcised men with a replacement foreskin through regenerative tissue technology.

has no effect, but deep down it all made sense because of what was missing.

However, even in that denial stage, I soon realized crying would get me nowhere. If anything, *I* would make it happen. I began cross taping and a couple months later bought a Dual Tension Restorer (DTR).[139] I began researching hours on male anatomy and found many, many similarities between men and women physiologically (especially when it came to sexual organs). I discovered things about male sexuality that I never imagined: prostate stimulation, multiple orgasms, dry orgasms; the list went on and on.

I also realized how important it is to discover other people's problems and help them fix them, be it relevant to you or not. It stings that it took something like this for me to realize that everyone needs a little help from the world, but it's better late than never. Whenever I can, I try to chip in something, be it lyme disease treatment or a new bridge for a small city to have faster transport to school. I knew the importance of education, but never was the duty to educate others so important to me. If my parents knew about this they would have never done it, and if I never knew about circumcision I would live the rest of my life trying to find what part of me was missing. And circumcision is just the tip of the iceberg—think of all the other things in life I never knew that could make me a better human being.

In short, my circumcision story had many more benefits than losses. Would it have been better if I had learned these life lessons and facts in another way? Of course. But if this is how I became a better man, then I will gladly accept it. My advice is to always look at everything with an open mind, question what you've been told, be honest and accepting with yourself, always strive for improvement and always remember how important it is to support others in their struggles. If it wasn't for the support I have received, I would never have gotten to where I am now.

Michael Gates
19 years
California, USA
12 January 2014

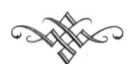

---

[139] The Dual Tension Restorer (DTR) is sold by www.foreskinrestore.com.

My Feelings About My Circumcision

In 1964 I was circumcised at birth by "well-meaning" parents who listened to the doctors of the day. It was done before I even left the hospital after I was born. Scarred for life, and not even 48 hours old. My father was actually out of town and not present when I was born. Therefore, I don't know if my parents had ever discussed the issue or if it was my mother's sole decision. If anyone gave permission, it was my mother.

Of course, in 1964, I don't know if the doctors even gave the parents much choice in the matter, either. I did ask my mother once, years later, and she was convinced that being cut was cleaner and healthier. This from a nurse. Fourteen years later, when my brother was born, he was subject to routine infant circumcision, as well. My father was present at the hospital for the birth. Brother came home circumcised. So I presume it was one of those things that was just done for him, too.

My father was cut at about eight years old, 1941/1942 time frame, so he presumably never knew what having a foreskin as an adult felt like. I asked him once. That means he never had sex as an adult with a foreskin. My paternal grandfather passed away when I was still young. I knew my maternal grandfather into my adulthood, but I never knew whether or not he was cut. I remember the skin on my father's penis as being "looser" fitting than mine. It also looms larger in my mind than what I have. I always wondered what that dark ring around my penis was.

Randomly looking at Amazon, somehow a search brought up Jim Bigelow's book, *The Joy of Uncircumcising*.[140] I bought it in printed form, and read it very quickly. It must have been about 1998, when I was 34. I have tried a lot of the various tugging methods since. Tried cross taping, a PUD, 12 or 16oz, off and on.[141] Taping was just so inconvenient for me. Never could "pee through" the hole in the PUD without making a mess.

Still watching the Internet, came across the O'Hara's book, *Sex as Nature Intended It*.[142] As a blow-in, there a reference to TUG-A-HOY, so I got one of

---

[140] Jim Bigelow, *The Joy of Uncircumcising!; Exploring Circumcision: History, Myths, Psychology, Restoration, Sexual Pleasure and Human Rights* (Aptos: Hourglass Publishing, 1992): 52.

[141] The PUD or Penile Uncircumcising Device was invented by Roland Clark and patented in 1996.

[142] Karen O'Hara & John O'Hara, *Sex As Nature Intended It* (Hudson: Turning Point, 2002)

those and used it till it broke.[143] Cleaned the house and got rid of the first copy of the book. Bought another one later which had a blow-in reference to the CAT line of foreskin restoration products.[144] Finally, I got some TLC Tuggers.[145] I am mostly covered when soft, but nowhere near covered when erect. Fifteen years of restoration, and who knows when I'll stop.

Why do we cut little boys like this? It seems so barbaric. My reaction to what I've learned about the spread and effects of circumcision is mostly sadness. According to what I've read, even the ancient Jewish culture was not so extreme as what is typically done in the US.

We are all victims of misguided people who have perpetuated a barbaric practice and continue to make excuses to justify it. For instance, circumcision as a "cure" for masturbation? Didn't work for me, any time I get the chance, I do.[146]

Ctrclckws
49 years
New York, USA
10 November 2013

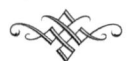

---

[143] The TUG-A-HOY is a tapeless foreskin restoration device invented by Dr James A. Haughey and patented in 2003.

[144] CAT is a Constant Applied Tension foreskin restoration device, available from www.catstretcher.com.

[145] TLC Tugger is a restoration device invented by Ron Low.

[146] Anecdotal accounts suggest that infant circumcision does prevent masturbation until puberty, which is the reason for the medical profession introducing infant circumcision in the late nineteenth century. Circumcision does not stop post-pubertal masturbation; in fact, research indicates that circumcised males tend to masturbate more frequently. See E.O. Laumann, C.M. Masi and E.W. Zuckerman, "Circumcision in the United States," *Journal of the American Medical Association* 277, 13 (1997): 1052-7.

My Surgical Foreskin Restoration

My mother told me the doctor circumcised me when I was nine days old, before I was able to consent, refuse, or even understand why the doctor was hurting my penis.

We were Catholic, so it wasn't done for religious reasons. In 1938 it was standard to keep mothers in the hospital for ten days, and to circumcise boys at about a week. After taking me home, my parents heard me crying that night, and they found my penis bleeding. The doctor came and put stitches into the frenular area, and the marks are visible today.

Unlike today, doctors did not inject local anesthesia for newborn circumcisions, or even administer Tylenol to take the edge off the pain. Mercifully, I have no memory of having been held down, struggling and crying, and I don't remember the burning pain of the scalpel severing my foreskin, or the snipping away of my inner lining and frenulum. I don't remember the post-operative pain, bleeding, or the sting of the needle inserting stitches. Nor do I remember the liquid fire of hot urine hitting the raw red glans and the open wound, the inevitable consequence of circumcision during infancy.

Why me? Why was I part of the unlucky 50% of boys that year in New York City circumcised at birth? Maybe it was just bad luck. Another, more sinister reason may have been related to something my mother kept telling me when I was a child. She'd said that I'd caused her a lot of pain during my birth, and perhaps she consented to have the end of my penis snipped off so that I would also feel pain. It might have been a form of retaliation.

This unnecessary mutilation has affected my entire life, and I grieved for my lost foreskin, eventually having it reconstructed by plastic surgery. I didn't know if I'd been born with a short or long one. I was tempted to think that I'd been born with a long, rubbery, nippled hood, generously proportioned to allow for erection and growth, but I will never know.

My mother told me that my "pee-pee" had been cut to make it cleaner. This had terrified me, and I anxiously compared my tiny trimmed weenie with my father's thick Italian sausage and saw that I lacked the prominent sleeve of thick skin over the tip. When I saw him urinate, I noted how he pulled the hood back to let the stream flow neatly and unobstructed from his tip. From the moment I saw that I was lacking what my father had, I felt that I'd never be the man he was.

I repeatedly tried to stretch my shaft-skin over the glans, to see what my penis would have looked like if it had not been cut. I'd pull my shaft-skin forward and it would bunch up to cover the head. The core of my cock would retract into my abdomen, leaving only a stubby end covered with skin. The instant I let go, it always snapped back hard to bare the glans totally, to my intense frustration. Covering the head with skin was possible only when my penis was soft; with erection the slack disappeared, and the skin would only cover the rim when I tugged hard.

Psychological Reactions

All during my childhood I never let on to anyone how much I grieved for my lost foreskin because I was too embarrassed to discuss my loss. Each time I saw a normal penis, it reminded me of what I'd lost even more vividly than the sight of the scar on mine. To console myself, by wishful thinking, I developed a theory that my foreskin would grow back later, based on my observation that all the older boys I'd seen had foreskins. I almost convinced myself this was true, as I'd seen many other features, such as facial hair and deepening of the voice that appeared with maturity.

At that early age, it was too frightening for me to accept that I'd been marked for life, and that my penis would never be whole again. The sight of the irregular brown scar ring behind my naked glans was a constant reminder of my violated body every time I urinated, undressed, or bathed. Never having been a conformist, I was not consoled because others were circumcised as well, and I wished for a normal, untrimmed penis. If there were only a single foreskin left in the world, I'd want it to be on my penis.

I enjoyed touching my penis, and soon learned the pleasures of making it grow hard. At this time I met Danny, a year older than me. I saw him make good use of his unspoiled gift from nature, because he proudly and joyfully masturbated in front of me several times. I tried to imitate him, but without a foreskin, I was unable even to make a start. I asked him why I couldn't do what he did. He inspected my penis and replied, "Yours has been cut." Apparently that was his entire knowledge about circumcision and its effects. It left me again lamenting my butchered penis, and I despaired of ever ejaculating.

Learning Different Strokes

My first successful masturbation was at age twelve, bumping my corona with the tight shaft skin, and this reassured me that I could do what I'd seen older boys do. It took me a long time to come, as my glans was dry and desensitized. With pubertal growth, my shaft-skin became tighter as the core of my cock outgrew it, and eventually became drumhead tight with erection. In effect, I had less skin to work with as I matured, and found it increasingly difficult to pull the skin up over my rim, which was why I turned to lubricants.

By the time I was sixteen, my erect penis was about six inches. I'd never been dissatisfied with what nature had given me, as I felt my dick's only deficiency was lack of a foreskin.

My tip (glans) was rim-sensitive instead of having the hot button underneath.[147] Perhaps this was because my frenulum had been amputated at birth, unlike some circumcised boys who had a thick strip of tissue running from the groove under the glans to meet the shaft-skin farther back, evidence that they hadn't been butchered as badly.[148] I'd also noticed that my brown scar ring was jagged and lopsided, more skin having been removed on the left side. Unlike some cut cocks I'd seen, mine had little or no inner lining left between the rim and the scar, only granular scar tissue that had filled the area where my nerve-rich inner lining had been removed. Despite this, the area between my rim and scar was very sensitive.

When I thought of what had been done to it without my consent, I felt that I'd been violated and abused, a feeling I later found was common among males who resented having been circumcised. I repeatedly wondered what it would feel like to have a snug sleeve of skin to run up and down my glans to bring orgasm as I'd seen natural boys do.

---

[147] The "rim" or corona of the glans is sensitive to fine touch.
[148] In the United States it is common practice to remove the highly sensitive frenulum along with the foreskin. This restricts the main sources of pleasurable sensory input to the desensitized glans corona and mucosal remnants.

Seeking Restoration

My envy of intact males became more intense, and every time I saw one, my wish for a foreskin increased. I'd read that several plastic surgeons had replaced foreskins for circumcised males. One had been done by a South African plastic surgeon, according to a 1963 article in the *British Journal of Plastic Surgery*.[149] I didn't have the money to fly to South Africa, so this prospect was tantalizingly out of reach. It's important to note that at the time, restoration by stretching the remaining skin was unknown, at least to me, and I thought plastic surgery was the only way to do it. Today, I would not make the same choice.

During my quest, I encountered others who resented their circumcisions. Those who felt strongly enough to seek restoration were very intense, and had harsh words about the doctors who had mutilated them. Several described their feelings as "rage," and I could easily sympathize with this.

The Surgery

I had plastic surgery to rebuild my foreskin when I was forty-three years old by a plastic surgeon who had done five others before me. Using general anesthesia, the surgeon cut a ring of shaft-skin free a couple of inches behind the head, inverting it over the glans to form the inner lining. This skin tube remained attached to my penis behind the glans to form the preputial sac.[150] He then put the re-covered glans into a slit in my scrotum, as his plan was to use scrotal skin to form the outer covering. He stitched it to the shaft-skin where he'd cut free the inner hood, and to the end of the inverted lining. This left the end of my penis buried in my scrotum, making me unable to have a full erection. He had done a poor job of suturing, leaving a gap at the cut line on my shaft. When I pointed this out to him, he said it would heal by granulation.

He'd also made the orifice too tight, and when I told him of this, he said he'd correct it later. This left a very small orifice for urination, and I was forced to sit down and dab the orifice with toilet paper afterward. This inconvenience was to continue, and I began to feel that he wasn't as competent as I'd hoped.

---

[149] Jack Penn, "Penile Reform," *British Journal of Plastic Surgery* 16 (1963): 287-88.

[150] The inner lining of the new foreskin (analogous in structure to the mucosa of a normal foreskin) formed the *preputial sac*.

More Complications

Three months after the first operation, the surgeon cut loose most of the scrotal skin, leaving my penis attached to my scrotum by a strip of skin about ¼ inch thick. He did not tie off the bleeders adequately, and the operative site was seeping blood after he'd finished. A massive hematoma[151] resulted, and the consequent scar contraction had made the orifice phimosed and my new hood totally unretractable.

Another complication was that healing formed adhesions between the inner and outer layers, preventing full retraction until I'd worked them loose. I sought to widen my hood's orifice to let it slip back easily over my glans, even with full erection. This is important for sex because bare glans contact during coital thrusting is much more satisfying than thrusting into a tight hood.

I had to do a lot of stretching because of my large glans. Hot baths helped, as the heat relaxed the scrotal graft covering the end of my penis, and helped me insert small segments of plastic tubing into the orifice and taping them in place as "spacers" to stretch my orifice. The main task was to insert the spacer, then tape it in place. Once the spacer was in place, it didn't matter if the hood tightened again. In fact it helped, as the spacer would stretch the ring muscle when it was fully contracted. I used progressively larger spacers as I progressed. Eventually, I was able to use a 35mm plastic film container as the orifice widened. That was about as large as I needed, and masturbation loosened my hood further.

It took a few years until my new hood was fully retractable during erection. The foreskin remained mostly over the glans, stimulating the entire head and giving me a bonus in sensation. Meanwhile, I still sat down to urinate, and often the orifice was so contracted that the hood ballooned out under the pressure of retained urine. Even after loosening my foreskin's orifice, I had to be careful urinating. Previously, I'd stood and relaxed my muscles to start the flow, but now I found this wasn't adequate. Unless I retracted my hood to expose the orifice, the stream would splatter uncontrollably.

After this second operation and its problems, I decided not to allow this surgeon to continue with his program of further surgery to "touch up" my penis, especially as he'd said it would take three more operations to complete the task. I'd had enough and was unwilling to take further risks. The outer layer of my new foreskin was made of scrotal skin, with a pebbly texture and darker color than my shaft-skin, and its hairs continued to grow. I'd heard

---

[151] *Hematoma* is a local accumulation of blood leaked from the blood vessels.

that electrolysis would remove these, but I'd never met anyone who'd had this done, which is why I didn't try it. Instead, I used an electric shaver, a simple and safe method. I never found any solution to the sharp contrast in skin tone and texture between my shaft-skin and the graft, although one person suggested tattooing the shaft-skin to match the graft.

The new hood remained insensitive for a couple of years, as nerves regenerate slowly. Eventually, I experienced sensation in my "foreskin," but it was not as sensitive or erotic as a natural foreskin would have been. An additional problem was that my new hood did not produce smegma, because my original inner lining, with its smegma-producing glands, had been completely removed.[152] I used cocoa butter to lubricate the hood and prevent irritation. I never overcame this deficiency, and today I still have to use lubricant to keep my penis-sleeve lubricated.

Rewards

Sensitivity returned quickly because I had complete glans coverage. Other patients had told me that sensitivity improves once the glans is re-hooded, but I was skeptical because I knew that much sexual "sensitivity" is in the brain. About three months after surgery, I turned over in bed one night, half-awake, and the end of my penis pushed from its shroud to touch the sheet, producing a feeling of tenderness in the glans. I realized then that the sensitivity was real, as this had not been a sexual setting.

Later, I encountered other evidence of increased glans sensitivity by comparing my experiences with others. Before restoration, I'd never felt irritation in my glans from contact with clothing. An uncut friend of mine had told me that when he had tried keeping his foreskin back, friction from clothing on his naked glans was unbearable. When I tried it, the feel of clothing against the head was uncomfortable. My satisfaction with the novel sensations provided by my new hood was profound. I enjoyed touching my penis, even in non-sexual situations, feeling the delicious sensations. One bonus was size. The scrotal graft was thicker than my shaft-skin, and the front part of my penis bulged because of my prominent glans. When I retracted it during erection, the thick hood locked back behind the flaring corona, filling the groove and forming a bulging collar around the shaft.

---

[152] It was once thought that human males produced smegma from glands, but such glands have yet to be identified.

On the negative side, I'd lost a lot of scrotal skin, and my balls were now tight against my body, instead of hanging freely as they had before. This worried me, because it sometimes appeared that I had no testicles at all, but eventually my scrotum stretched somewhat.

My Sexual Re-Birth

Restoration gave me a sexual re-birth, a profound physical and psychological experience, and I felt an urgent need to masturbate to catch up on sensations denied me during my early years. Post-operative soreness after the hematoma had healed was erotic because it made me more aware of my penis between sexual episodes, and I greatly enjoyed my new consciousness. Every time I touched my penis I felt a twinge of pain as the scar tissue stretched, reminding me of my reshaped state. With more sensitivity, I enjoyed a new dimension in sex. I could now relax because my newly increased sensitivity allowed me to stimulate my penis gently, and let the fulfilling sensations of orgasm come to me.

I tried other lubricants, including Vitamin E oil and K-Y Jelly thinned with water. I liked the wet, slippery sensations of K-Y best, because I enjoyed the feeling of my copiously lubricated glans slipping around inside my foreskin whenever I moved. However, because K-Y was water-based, it tended to absorb residual urine and quickly developed an unpleasant odor. Still, various lubricants enabled me to try different sensations. Natural lubricant would come during fantasizing.

In 1987, a man who had restored his foreskin by stretching told me about Retin-A cream, a prescription cream used for mild chemical abrasion. The mucous surface of the circumcised glans thickens as it dries, and becomes ten times thicker.[153] I used Retin-A to remove the outer hardened layers, dead cells that masked my sensations. This also freshened the inverted shaft-skin that made up the inner surface of my hood. I saw the surface of my glans becoming smoother and glossier after several treatments.

---

[153] It is a common belief that the glans surface (mucosa) becomes more thickened (keratinized) as a result of circumcision. One study found no difference, see Dinh M.H. et al. "Keratinization of the adult male foreskin and implications for male circumcision" *AIDS* 24, 6 (2010): 899-906.

Summing Up

I am more or less happy with what I have, based on the idea that half a loaf is better than none. I cannot get back all the nerve endings lost when the doctor cut off my foreskin and frenulum, but my glans is more sensitive than before, and sex is much more enjoyable now.

Would I do it over again? Yes, but not by surgery, which was very unsatisfactory because of the complications and because it left scars. A doctor had caused the original problem, and putting myself and my penis in the hands of another doctor was foolish. Instead, I would do it by stretching, as many have done since I had my surgery.

Jack Santoro
75 years
New Mexico, USA
25 October 2013

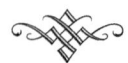

Oregon Intactivist

I was fifteen when I had to have surgery and, while I was under, the doctor circumcised me, because it's "cleaner" and all the other false reasons they give.

When I woke up, I immediately threw up from the pain and then looked under the covers and saw I had stitches where nobody wants stitches. I then proceeded to throw up again from the sight of what had been done to me.

As soon as I healed, I knew my life had changed forever. I had far less foreskin, a remnant of my frenulum left (that registered no feeling), and nothing was lined back up correctly. Erections were painful, my glans was out of shape from being pulled down too tight, and there was a bend to the left I had never had.

Fast forward some years and sex was OK, but it certainly was not the mind-blowing experience I had heard about. As a matter of fact, I remember thinking, "Is this what everybody was talking about?" Since being married, my wife has enjoyed the sex more than I ever did.

I can't begin to describe the pain and the heartache being circumcised has caused me over the years. However, I can tell you from personal experience: A circumcised penis is not what we as men were intended to have. Do your son a favor and leave him whole. Circumcision doesn't just hurt physically or just infants, it hurts men too. We need to speak out against this practice.

There has been some good that came out of this, and that is I left both of my boys intact, so they could experience sex as it is intended some day. I did discover restoration and have had good results.

James31254[154]
41 years
Oregon, USA
25 September 2013

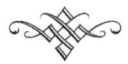

___
[154] http://oregonintactivist.com/circumcision-stories/oregon-intactivist/ (accessed 25 September 2013). Used with permission.

Parental Denial

My relationship with my parents has been practically non-existent since I told them how I felt. It all happened within the first couple of weeks after I discovered the truth about circumcision, the foreskin, and the whole nine yards.

I hate to get all sappy and dramatic, but I don't think I'd be exaggerating if I said that at that particular point in my life I had never felt more hopeless, helpless, and useless. I was at my wit's end and my emotional rock bottom. So, it wasn't a question of "if" but "when" I'd tell my parents how I felt. And, when I finally did, my dad hardly blinked before he literally called me an idiot and told me: "This is America, everybody does it!"

Of course, I'd tell him that about eighty-five percent of the world *doesn't* "do it" and that America probably has one of the largest percentages of sexual dysfunction in the world.

His response? "Eighty-five percent of the world lives in the dirt! You need to go to a shrink or something because there's *nothing wrong with you.*" He also couldn't wait to tell me that "all the porno guys are circumcised" and how he and his younger brother constantly mocked my uncle (who was born in Germany and intact) for having a "German weenie." As if *any* of this shallow, trivial, childish nonsense would somehow sway me or comfort me in any way.

Sure, he was just trying to comfort me—I could tell myself that, but I know better. I know deep down that's not what he was trying to do. He's too petty a person for that. He's a simpleton and I can see right through everything he does, like he was a bad comic relief character in a stage production. None of that elaborate hodgepodge of clichés, hearsay, blanket statements, and racism was for me. It was all just part of an elaborate shield for his own ego. The fact that he would have such utter disregard for me, even when I was literally at my emotional rock bottom, infuriates me to absolutely no end.

My mother, a nurse, was maybe slightly more receptive upon my revelation but still very, very stubborn. Naturally, a mother doesn't want to outright admit that she hurt her only child, so she was simply trying to cover herself. That doesn't excuse her behavior (nor does it excuse her calling my dad in to gang up on me), but if you look at it from that perspective, at least it makes sense. Nowadays, the topic doesn't come up much, but when it does, she's much more understanding and receptive to my comments about the issue and seems to acknowledge what was partly her mistake (although she still doesn't seem to fully comprehend and/or recognize the degree to which people are affected by this operation). So, I can't say I have much of a qualm with her anymore.

My dad, however, will never apologize for all of the physical and emotional pain he's caused me because it's simply not in him. Any subsequent time (the occurrence of which has been very rare, thankfully) the subject comes up, his reaction is just different degrees of the same. So fuck it, I don't bring it up. But even then, the damage is done. Any trust in him or admiration for him I once had is gone. I'll never forgive him for as long as I live.

Anyway, enough of that. Things are rough right now and restoration has been kind of a pain to get rolling, but believe it or not, I feel optimistic, so maybe I'll find my "happy place" and get over it some day.

TopHat
19 years
Virginia, USA
24 May 2010

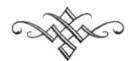

Problem With No Name

My mother was a nurse. When I was born, nearly all babies in the USA were circumcised. Mother wanted a tight circumcision—total—so I wouldn't "do something disgusting like touch myself." Apparently baby boys do that even in the crib. So from the beginning she knew that touching oneself was pleasurable with a foreskin and, if you ablated the parts that felt good, then no more pleasure and no problem (for her). I asked her late in life if she would have done the same to a daughter and she said "No, they don't do that, but girls aren't 'disgusting' like boys."

Like most boys, however, I did "touch myself" but found early on that I needed lotion. Ironically enough, I found my mother's hand lotions! Without the lotion, it was rough and chafed—I could still masturbate but needed to get some semen out as lotion. Otherwise, forget it. By age forty, sex was impossible without lotion.

My first experience of sex with a woman on a regular and sober basis was in my late twenties. I could not get off with oral sex—not enough friction. My ex-wife had had an intact husband prior and he enjoyed stroking of hand and mouth enormously. But I felt nothing. However, she came from a family line of mohels[155] and was pleased with the look of my penis and the fact that it was a clean, total cut. Still, we both agreed that if we had boys (we didn't— we had girls) they would not be circumcised, because it is a barbaric genital mutilation. And, she knew first hand (literally!) that it greatly reduced a man's pleasure. What mother would wish that on her son?

Our sex life was good enough at the beginning of our twenty-year marriage. But as time passed, by age thirty and certainly by age forty, there was too little sensation in my penis to feel much during intercourse. Oral sex was never possible and that left me finishing myself with my hand after she had her multiple orgasms with oral sex. Not very sexy—masturbating after pleasing your woman.

During our marriage, the gender difference in sexual pleasure was a real source of tension. I knew that naturally women enjoyed sex way more than men. She would always have more than one orgasm and they were earthshaking. I never had an earthquaking orgasm or more than one because of the male refractory period. But then, the fact that I am a man born into a genital cutting society meant I knew my penis was getting weaker every year.

---

[155] A *mohel* is a Jewish ritual circumciser.

By the time I neared fifty I had lost interest in even masturbating. Well, the interest was there but it took too much effort to get the remnant of frenulum not eroded with time to feel anything. I used to joke, half kiddingly, that I wish I had female genitalia because the doctors would leave it alone. Plus, we both knew women enjoyed sex so much more, but to rob me of the pleasure a man can have created not grief but anger at the whole Abrahamic tradition of genital cutting. What type of God makes it his covenant to cut off penis nerve endings?[156] Then believers conquer unbelievers and offer their conquered foreskins as a holocaust to God?[157]

Long story short, for the past ten years of our marriage intercourse was a chore. I had to really concentrate on some fantasy, stroke myself to the edge before penetration, then keep focused on the little pleasure that was there. A woman enjoys not only being pleased but pleasing her man. It was obvious that she couldn't please me—not her fault but my circumcised anatomy. So one thing that brought us together, at least in the beginning, became a source of tension.

After the divorce, the last thing I thought of was sex with a woman. I have strong full erections. My health is excellent (BMI perfect, exercise daily), but the strong erection conceals the fact that there are few nerve endings left. At fifty I am a strong healthy man with a dead penis. A girlfriend could stroke it and stroke it and "How does that feel?" Well, it doesn't. So I would simply please and not be pleased. The lack of reciprocity and give and take is really damaging to a man-woman relationship. And my dry penis would hurt her and what man wants to hurt the woman he loves for—maybe, maybe!—three seconds of pleasure and no buildup at all?

The lack of buildup was the thing that made all sexual encounters in our marriage so poor. She would build up and enjoy again and again. So, I would spend an hour or two in an erect state but no buildup. Eventually, although I was willing to give and not receive, my ex-wife tired of it and viewed our lovemaking as separate masturbation sessions (which they were, really). So we stopped having sex, she got a vibrator, and I retreated to the bathroom for occasional release of semen to eliminate discomfort.

The first thing my ex-wife said to a new girlfriend was "Sex with him will be

---

[156] Scholars assert that the covenant is more priestly than divine. Thirteen centuries after Abraham's lifetime, the priests of the second temple inserted the instruction for the mandatory circumcision of infants into the *Torah* as Genesis 17. See Leonard B. Glick, *Marked in Your Flesh: Circumcision from Ancient Judea to Modern America* (York: Oxford University Press, 2005), 15-6.

[157] The Slaughter of the Shechemites, Genesis 34.

lousy. He can feel nothing and his dry hard penis will hurt you." Whoa! She knows why it is dry and hard but would literally rub it in the face of other women, telling them to choose a man who was intact.

The whole experience from my mother to my ex-wife left me very bitter. But to complain about the lack of sensation worsened relations with the wife. "Real men don't complain."

No, we just suffer terribly from this "problem with no name."

John
51 years
Illinois, USA
12 December 2013

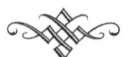

Questioning

I am getting so depressed about my circumcision. Subconsciously, it is an issue I always knew was there. Having studied what has happened to me and hearing from men and women, I am just getting so depressed. My life is not ruined. Maybe I am even one of the more lucky ones. Yet I am still depressed. Who had the right to do this to me? Are not my genitals my own? Nature made men and women to match and someone, some selfish insensitive jerk, robbed me of this match for a mere 400 or so dollars. I hope he suffers sharp fire of correction.

I will feel much better in myself when I don't feel inferior to others. I don't know how I can't feel sexually inferior for loss of function, and if not for that, at least for the pain and soreness I sometimes feel. I do feel inferior to foreign men in general, and intact American men. I think they are different in profound and subtle ways physically and emotionally. I think they are more sensual and natural, and have less trauma. They still may have been traumatized, though, and can still commit great acts of evil. But pain in all forms begets pain. Hurt people hurt people, and traumas perpetuate traumas. I really do envy intact men and not just for their foreskin, but for the experience they got in life that we did not—a more wholesome family life. Less depression.

The circumcision trauma is probably the deepest, most hidden, and most painful, and yet it is probably not alone by itself. The other later traumas and issues (and we all have them no matter how we deny them) probably had their roots at least in part in the circumcision trauma. Original traumas and losses often beget other traumas and losses, or exacerbate them, making them more intense.

What the hell is wrong with the medical profession? What the hell is wrong with society? What gives society, or parents, or the doctors the right to think they can do this? Is it any wonder I feel used when I learn that they sell my most precious body part for cosmetic uses to make a huge profit? They profit off pain and misery and the destruction of sexuality and even the family, all for a little money and for people's vanity! It makes me cry inside that they sold my foreskin for profit. Did they even tell my parents? I certainly will. I already have been losing respect for medicine, but this takes the cake. They do not seem to me to really care about health or ethics. What's more, they want not only our money but also our respect! Why are we paying these masters to lord over us? We should try to take health into our own hands as much as possible.

Now that I learn how doctors have to forcibly pull the foreskin away from the glans, it makes me wonder how they even decided this was a worthy operation. That fact alone would cause a rational man to hesitate in the procedure, but not those who are seeking profit, are upholding tradition or religious beliefs, or are just plain psycho. Circumcising doctors are sociopaths in my opinion. No wonder the world criticizes American men, I think. They don't understand our trauma.

I believe that a child can feel pain even right after it is just born. I mean, who cannot believe this? Only the idiots who want to justify their harmful practices. This should be so obvious.

But I go farther. I believe that children can even feel things like humiliation and indignation. So I believe that when a boy is laying on the operating table after the surgery, *totally objectified and exposed*, he is probably internalizing his status as a man. He is probably suffering humiliation and shame. Things that I understood intellectually I now understand with immediate clarity and perception. I can now visualize the doctor doing it to me—in part—by having watched a video online.

I think the body keeps a record of all the memories and feelings it has ever had. The feeling or bodily memory transcends words and abstractions, goes deeper, and is more primal than cognitive memory. A little serious pain and suffering at a later stage doesn't do much harm. But I believe that this sort of pain (and loss) at this sort of age and time is highly traumatic—plus we bear a permanent reminder of it. Plus, I occasionally suffer soreness after orgasm or friction that extends all the way down to the bottom of my body, near my anus. It is not pleasant. Thanks, Doc.

I think a lot of people who get circumcised live their lives in denial. That is the saddest. Better they learn about what happened, deal with it, process it, grieve about it, use it as a chance to connect with a deeper part of themselves and others. But denial only produces pathological behavior. Because I write this and talk about this with others, I am somewhat freed from pathological behavior. But, I am not freed from depression.

This goes in levels. I will process some, write about some of my feelings, then I will sleep and wake and converse, remember and forget, and then process more. Most people can't handle the truth or can't handle a man's pain. They pretend to be interested in a woman's pain, but they are only seeking to validate their weak male ego.

My parents don't want to hear about my circumcision. And sometimes I feel like being a good little boy who doesn't bother them or rub this mistake in their faces. But I know that is not good for dealing with grief. I know that cowardice doesn't help anything, not when I have an honest emotion to share. I also imagine that my father's circumcision has negatively impacted my parents' sex life, hence their bond, hence our childhood through that way. They get along mostly well but there is some tension and lack of passion. Could foreskin have anything to do with that? My dad won't restore; he said he's fine. Damn, I am just as politically conservative as him but he's conservative in a stupid way as well.

I want to talk about it, especially when it makes people feel awkward. My desire is that my parents should feel depressed about what she did. Why should they not feel depressed? I would be so happy if my mother had a permanently broken heart because of it. Maybe she does, but then I hope she would be conscious of it and able to share her feelings. My mother cannot share her feelings very well, so she resorts to shaming and blaming, and histrionics.

Why can't I just forgive them and forget about it? I won't stop till I get to the very very bottom of my depression. Until I have woken my family up, circumcised all of their hearts completely. I'm not saying I'll succeed. I'm only saying I won't stop. I can't change people, but I can make sure they understand my position and have my voice in their head, if they want to have a relationship with me.

Women keep telling me how sex is different, better with intact men. It hurts but I need to know the pain, because you are only bringing up to my higher mind what my lower mind already knows. Keep telling me how much you like intact cock. Keep telling me the truth, for the truth shall set me free. Interestingly my ex-girlfriend thought this. I had a few sexual problems with her—although great sex overall, or pretty good sex. At least I gave her orgasms. Clitoral ones. OK, I can now see how she and our relationship were wounded by my circumcision. It is my desire to contact her and maybe we can restore our relationship or maybe not, but at least find a deeper connection. She wishes I was more in the body, enjoying myself in life. I wonder how many misdiagnoses, confusions, blaming statements and judgments have happened between lovers and couples because of what an idiot surgeon did.

They cut our bodies and wounded our flesh, and that affects our soul on a deep level. But the cut did not actually enter the soul. We can regrow our souls as we regrow our foreskin, although this can be even more complete. In fact it can be made beyond what was taken—like a tree that was pruned, it can grow even better. We can just ignore and deny what has happened and become criminals, sociopaths, aggressive angry men, or passive men going their own way, but that is a choice we make, not what the doctor made for us. But our souls or spirits are not wounded. They may actually grow. And yet I can't deny that when circumcised and when one deals with the trauma and loss, it does seem to spiritualize one. Or is spiritualizing oneself a pathology, a sign of anti-sensuality and anti-life?

I'm a Christian and now I am struggling with the God of the Old Testament —why he would require it of Israel's children. That doesn't make any sense, so now I struggle with faith issues. I understand Abraham circumcised himself as a sign of a covenant. I wonder what Sarah thought about that. And yet at least that was done as an adult with his knowledge.

To have it done to children? That doesn't sound like God, but who am I to question the potter? I guess Christ was crucified on the cross. I guess he suffered more. Plus he was circumcised. But I wonder why God commanded Abraham to do it?[158] It was a commandment that had to do with circumcision of the heart. Lo and behold, I do find it has led to greater circumcision of my heart. But anyway that's over; that was put an end to. Paul says circumcision profits nothing.[159] God forbid I would circumcise my own son, out of a desire that he experience what I did. What kind of man would I be for that? I am glad I am thinking about this now.

I came to the conclusion that there is the natural path a boy is put on when he is born. It is a much easier, much more sensual and automatic path towards life's ends, joys, relationships, and fulfillment. Lucky bastards. Now, when we are cut, at whatever age, but especially as a powerless child, we are put on a second path. That path can also lead to joy and fulfillment, but there are so many more obstacles, and so much grief has to be gone through. Maybe it spiritualizes us a bit, to the extent that any trauma and loss can spiritualize someone. I don't say this as a justification. God wanted to spiritualize Israel as they were a chosen nation, but I object to the fact that it was done to babies. No wonder they often rebelled against God.

I am just a man, with a limited physical body. I have no power save what the spirit gives me. Whatever works the spirit wants to do through me, that's all I can do. When I don't have the spirit, I don't have power. Flesh has only so

---

[158] Scholars assert that the priests of the second temple inserted the instruction for the mandatory circumcision of infants into into Genesis 17. See Leonard B. Glick, *Marked in Your Flesh: Circumcision from Ancient Judea to Modern America* (York: Oxford University Press, 2005), 15-6.

[159] "Circumcision is nothing and uncircumcision is nothing, but keeping the commandments of God." *Bible*, King James Version, I Corinthians 7:19.

much power. Everything great I have done has been without thinking, without my conscious will. I only want to be a temple of the Holy Spirit—what an honor.

See how this issue of circumcision is allowing me to see more clearly and come to terms with other issues? Jesus said that the greatest among you must be servants of all. That's how the heavenly hierarchy works. But on earth people are going around wanting to be masters of others, rich and famous and powerful and glorified. I tell you the truth, if there is any truth to the Bible or the afterlife, that we, if we continue in the grieving and healing process, we are the ones who are going to be glorified, and these people are going to be shamed.

I guess when I am in the spirit I don't feel the pain of my cut. I guess maybe due to this cut I may be in the spirit more. That could be a blessing. I wonder if there is a link here.

To get beneath all of these affects and emotions is a richly rewarding and powerful experience, with a ripple effect of benefits socially and personally. I find that to be true and I have only just started. Circumcision trauma and loss is really one of the deepest if not the deepest trauma and loss in my life. Cat Steven's song was right: "The first cut is the deepest." Dealing with other painful emotions has helped prepare me for this, but now it's time to go straight towards the center—and take down the medical establishment in the process. I am provoked. They asked for it: they awakened the beast.

But I also wonder about anger issues and such. I have minimized these in myself but every little thing has a cause. Occasionally I have had violent thoughts in my mind, or just generalized anger or anxiety about nothing in particular, for example, while walking down the street. Where do these issues come from? Certainly not completely from circumcision. From issues related to deep effects. I don't say it's all about childhood, but I say it is all about deep effects and implicit memories and repressed cognitive memories. That is why learning about this circumcision issue as a deep issue is so helpful.

It's time also to address my envy and self-image. I have envied intact men. I have slept around in the past with a few foreign women. They didn't say anything but I really wonder if they were thinking it. I would have appreciated them saying it, so then I could have started the process earlier. Only when in my late twenties as I started to do other emotional work did this idea start coming to my mind of its own accord without reading any other book or work about it or hearing about it, aside from Sam Keen's *Fire in the Belly*.[160] I still can't remember what he says about genital male mutilation, though I've read the book two or three times and I remember other parts of the book very well. That alone is interesting, is telling.

I will be better when I go to the deepest of my depths. It is important for me to be able to see and perceive the truth with clear eyes. It is important for me to be able to know automatically the difference between me and intact men. It is important for me to know what they have that I don't, so that I can account and adjust for their different attitudes and experiences. They must feel like kings and princes. I feel like a fool sometimes.

I will restore once I get the equipment and once I get more knowledge. I will never get my ridged band back, or my pheromone sources or estrogen receptors. I would like to learn more about them, but I will in good time. That makes me really sad. I am very excited about starting restoring. But that doesn't excuse those assholes, nor does it mean I shouldn't be depressed or envious. It is just so fucking not fair. Unfair. I know life is not fair, but come on! I mean, cutting off the most sensitive part of a man's body, his birthright, is worse than going through life poor. I'd rather have my foreskin than a million dollars.

I have a long way to go. Somehow I have to turn this trauma and loss into a gain. To me it's more of a loss than a trauma. What shape or form that gain may take is beyond me. Certainly I will grow back what I can. I can get the gliding function back, I think. That will make sex more enjoyable for both of us; it will cover the glans and there will be dekeratinization.[161] That will make it more enjoyable for me. No wonder masturbation hurt. My ex-girlfriend thought I was just a sexual prude.

I am single but I want to marry and take on a husband's responsibility. I am looking for a wife of good character. I am hoping my wife will be as distressed about this as I am. I hope to bring order in my life in terms of work, self-wellness, family and community relationships, my plan for future children, and in terms of social work that I want to do. Coming to an understanding of circumcision will help me deal with all this on all these levels. With the family it will open avenues that need to be opened. It will help me connect emotionally to people who always want to intellectualize and be abstract.

I believe I must find a way to make this turn out for the better somehow.

---

[160] Sam Keen, *Fire in the Belly* (New York: Bantam, 1991).
[161] *Dekeratinization* is the term used for the shedding of the outer callus tissue from the circumcised glans.

Since I lost so much, I must gain that much—even more if possible. That's the rule I go by in life. It keeps me sane, it keeps me satisfied and optimistic and hopeful about the future. It preserves my self-respect and my good mood. So how can I make something better come out of this? I often have no idea, but nature and life finds a way. I am not sure I will even experience that blessing in this life.

I have more to say and do. There is always more. I am probably not even ten percent finished externalizing my grief, and I will not be finished speaking until childhood circumcision is illegal everywhere.

Swordofpeace[162]
30 years
USA
4-6 June 2012

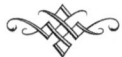

---

[162]Swordofpeace's contributon was edited from two web posts.

Restoration Works Brilliantly

I was circumcised as an infant in 1953. My childhood was pretty typical. I do not recall any incidents related to circumcision or foreskins except for one. My best friend in grade school was also my next-door neighbor, and we spent a lot of time together. I had ample time to see his penis, but never thought anything of it, except on one occasion that I can recall, when I told him his penis was not normal, though I do not remember the exact words I used. He retorted that maybe mine was not the normal one. Good life lesson that. But that short conversation was the extent of it.

I was the oldest of six children. My two younger brothers remained intact. As far as I know, that was never an issue, and the only time it came up was when I was in high school, I think, and I remember asking my mother why I was circumcised and not them. She answered that when I was born, the doctors recommended it and when my brothers were born the doctors did not. That satisfied me and I do not remember anything else on this issue.

I went to college and got a job as a scientist and found my strengths were big picture thinking, logic, and creatively finding solutions to problems. I do not remember any thoughts regarding being circumcised from this period, other than occasionally thinking it would be nicer to have a foreskin so I could go without underwear at times and not have my glans rub against my clothes and cause an erection.

After I got married and my wife was pregnant with our first child, I found that I had very strong feelings that if we had a son he should stay intact. Since I did not have any information about the value of foreskins, other than being more natural, this was surprising to me. My wife was happy to yield to my feelings on the matter, as she had not thought about it much and simply believed it to be something that was done routinely, presumably for good reasons.

Her gynecologist seemed fine with our decision to leave our son intact during our office visits. Then, at the birth, he went into an emotional rant, trying to convince me that our son would be traumatized by having a foreskin when I did not.[163] And while his ranting and emotional pleas did shake my resolve quite a bit and give me doubts about my choice to leave him intact, the total lack of logic in his argument was obvious, and I

---

[163] Circumcised doctors are more likely to push circumcision and have circumcised sons. See Andries J. Muller, "To cut or not to cut? Personal factors influence primary care physicians' position on elective newborn circumcision," *Journal of Men's Health* 7, 3 (2010): 227-232.

managed to resist his pleas.

I did not think much about foreskins again (other than learning to care for a boy with a foreskin and learning that many did not know how to do this) until one day, in 2001. I was at home bored, convalescing from surgery, and the Internet was just getting to a useful stage for research. On a whim, I looked up "foreskin restoration," expecting to see some plastic surgery discussion, perhaps. Instead I came upon several pages that discussed the value of foreskins, the horror of routine infant circumcision (RIC), and the possibility of nonsurgical restoration. For over an hour I literally could not stop reading, and when I was done, I knew that I had to try restoring.

I was blown away by my feelings of needing to do this. I did not expect much to come of it other than looking whole and natural, but that itself was, curiously, a very strong desire. And I do remember thinking that the descriptions of sexual improvements were way very much exaggerated. Analogies like "black and white TV compared to color TV" or "hearing a whole symphony versus a single instrument" seemed wildly embellished and unrealistic. For me, sex felt like the best and most amazing thing in the world, so it was inconceivable that it could be much better.

I immediately shared this information with my wife, who listened politely, then said she was worried that I would damage my penis, making sex less pleasurable. After some discussion and my reassuring her that I would be cautious and that I was compelled strongly to at least test the waters, I went back to research on the way to do this. I began with cross tape for a few days, then quickly switched to the pill tube method.

After a few days of that (and one minor skin tear) I realized that I could achieve the same thing without the pill tube. I quickly devised an alternative to t-tape, called t-tape strips and insert.[164]

As I slowly grew skin, I continued to gather information online, becoming a member of various list serves and forums that were available to discuss the value of foreskin, the horror of RIC, and related topics. Not only did this help keep me motivated, but it also gave me the chance to review and contribute to discussions and debates. I also began saving posts and articles that were particularly helpful, for future reference. After a while, I was asked to participate on several forums as a moderator.

Of course, staying motivated is only worthwhile if you get results. I can report that the results have dramatically exceeded my expectations. I can

---

[164] http://www.restoringforeskin.org/images/greg_b-t-tape-strips-and-insert-llustrated.pdf

report that you begin reaping the benefits sooner than you might think. In fact, my wife, who simply hoped I would not cause any negative effects, was the first to remark on how much better things felt during intercourse. This was just a month or so into my restoration. While neither of us could put a finger on what was better, the only reasonable explanation was the increased amount of skin. I should point out that I was left with very little inner skin (no coverage when flaccid, maybe ¼ inch left) and no skin movement when erect.

As time went on I grew more skin and the feelings became better and better. Around the four-month mark, sex and masturbation were becoming easy again. By that I mean to say that as a circumcised guy in my forties, I was having trouble in reaching climax.[165] I frequently had to take a rest part way through, and if I did not think of a good juicy fantasy to concentrate on, it was just not happening. I chalked this up to getting older and out of shape at the time.

But by four months into restoration, it was easy again, and getting to climax was like rolling off a log. I found that I was forgetting to think of fantasies. Amazing! Like setting the clock back to my twenties. Not only that, but, before, my wife could barely keep a hand job interesting for a few minutes, let alone bring me to climax. Now she easily brings me to climax, and she can play with different movements and techniques.

As I gained skin and experience, I learned a lot about what is needed to grow skin effectively. I learned how to avoid slow and no growth periods (keep tension level optimal), how to measure progress, and many other details. Restoration is simple in theory, but the details are very important. My training and experience in science probably helped greatly with this. If I were starting again today, I would make much faster progress than I was able to back then.

---

[165] This account confirms the anecdotal evidence that men circumcised in infancy notice a decline in penile sensitivity during their forties.

Seven years into my restoration, I began to experience whole body orgasms. This was new and I was totally unprepared for it. This seemed to be caused by unique feelings I had never experienced. They totally blew me away. And, to my surprise, I began to sound like those guys so long ago who seemed to be wildly exaggerating the sexual improvements that a foreskin provided. Now I was saying that it was like black and white versus color, or listening to a single instrument versus an orchestra. Even though my previous climaxes had always felt like the best feeling imaginable, this was so much better that they now seemed like a lackluster feeling that was hardly enough to remark on.

As I gained more experience (and orgasms became more intense and consistent), I began to realize that my climax was now very similar to what I saw my wife having. I traded notes with her, and we agreed that we seemed to be experiencing very similar climaxes.

But it is very hard to describe a climax, let alone how it has changed for me. Before, climax was the goal, everything leading up to it was to be rushed through to get to climax. At climax, my whole body tensed up, then released with several waves of contractions centered in my groin area. Afterward, though I needed to rest a bit, I could go again and repeat this sequence as many times as I wanted. Getting to climax was a precise dance that needed good focus, a good fantasy, and had to be done correctly in order to achieve climax.

Now, I do not need to fantasize. I am free to explore all sorts of variations. The feelings leading up to climax are so good that I enjoy tarrying and exploring along the way. Now the climax just happens: I do not need to focus or be precise. And as I get closer, the feelings just get better and better, until finally, my whole body convulses over and over. I am totally lost in it and have no control of my body, until after what feels like a long time. Then the convulsions slowly fade, and I find myself spent, barely able to move, feeling wonderful.[166]

---

[166] These are the orgasm types 2 and 3 as described by Kinsey et al. After a few years restoring, these "full body orgasms" can start to appear. Most circumcised men probably only ever experience type 1, which is basically just ejaculation without bodily sensation and involuntary movements. See Kinsey, A.C., Pomeroy, W.B. and Martin, C.E., *Sexual Behavior in the Human Male* (Philadelphia, PA: W.B. Saunders, 1948): 159-1.

Knowing how good sex should feel now, I firmly believe that the unspoken —but real—reason it is done to infants is this: If they had done this to grown men who had previously experienced whole body climaxes, the doctors would have been tarred and feathered—probably far worse—back when circumcision was first being promoted.

I am so grateful that I found out about restoration and the value of foreskins. We are so lucky that we can restore so much of the function and feeling by restoring. And I can say that restoration is well worth every second that it takes. As circumcised men, we are amputees who are missing critically important body parts. Restoration allows us to recover much of the function and feeling that was taken from us.

Greg B
61 years
Delaware, USA
6 October 2013

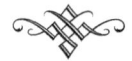

Restoring In A Predominately Intact Society

I was circumcised as an infant in 1945, and grew up in London. About a third of my classmates were cut, so different penises didn't bother me. I did the usual sports and athletics, even during the three years I spent in the army where communal showers/baths were the norm. I did have some fun playing with a schoolmate's intact penis several times but we soon grew out of that phase. It probably lasted about a year till I was thirteen years old or so. Many of my school pals did the same as we explored our developing bodies.

I did not ask my parents why I had been circumcised because my dad died when I was eleven and my mum in 1998, long before I discovered the Internet in 2010. I didn't realize my penis sensitivity was going to be a problem, or indeed that I'd missed out on about 50% of my sexual pleasure.

Twenty or so years ago, I saw a medical program on TV where a doctor explained how he had restored his penis but didn't go into detail about how he had accomplished this miraculous transformation. I set about doing the same, but there was no information back then. Over the following years, I slowly became frustrated and angry because of the time it took to make very little gains, but I tried to restore intermittently until, thanks to the Internet, I found out that I wasn't the only person trying to fashion a foreskin. This was three years ago and thanks to RestoringForeskin.org, I have made some good progress and found out quite a lot about how being cut has affected my life and the lives of my fellows.

I have given up wondering or being bothered about whether I am a latent gay and, even if there was such a thing, I feel sure that I would have had encounters with men at various times before now. I sometimes wonder if I am in love with myself—quite normal I think. I believe that being cut, as I am, has everything to do with how I feel about myself, and development of my private thought life. I am not bitter or angry with my late parents, as it was fairly normal to circumcise after the war and that, for me, was a long time ago.

I am not restored yet. I was a CI-4 last Christmas, but losing so much skin for so many months this year has set me back at least half a level. I couldn't restore properly for seven months. I'm very frustrated, though, because of the damage I occasionally do to my penis in restoring, and the time it takes to make any sort of progress. I will carry on restoring until either my penis or I give out.

The Chimera
68 years
London, England
27 October 2013

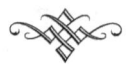

Restoring: Not Just For The Look Of It

I first remember hearing about a foreskin during one of my religion classes as a young boy. I remember that I had no idea what it was, but that it was something unnecessary that was cut off because God said to do it. I was always a curious child, though, and after thinking about it for a few days I dug through my mother's nursing manuals until I found an entry that described the foreskin: where it was, what it was, what it did, and all about its removal.

I looked at the pictures of the intact versus circumcised penis and I realized that I had been cut. I was horrified. My parents had allowed some doctor to cut mine off? They never even asked me if it was what I wanted. As I looked at the uncircumcised penis I thought it looked much better and I wished mine could look like that somehow. I was curious about my circumcision, though, and I asked my mother about it. She simply stated that it was done when I was born because of tradition (familial and religious). I wasn't happy with the response, but I was still only a child and was not about to yell at my mother because I was upset about something that happened when I was so little that I could not remember it.

As I grew older I heard jokes about intact guys, and it always made me feel bad. That they were being made fun of for something natural, something I wished I still had, angered me. I felt like part of me was missing and I could never get it back. In a way I almost envied the guys who got teased because at least they still had their foreskins.

When I hit puberty and began getting full erections I realized two things—it was fun to touch my penis, but when it got hard it was painful because of how tight the skin was. My circumcision had left me with barely enough skin to maintain an erection, but it was mildly painful and masturbation was not much fun once I got fully hard.

As a high-school student I thought this was just how things were going to be for the rest of my life until one day while I was searching for more information on foreskins and painful erections. I ran across a website that mentioned foreskin restoration, so I began to research it. I was scared about trying it, but at the same time, I was excited because it gave me hope that I might some day actually enjoy sexual pleasure, and perhaps have the beautiful look of an uncut penis.

I didn't start restoring until after I had joined the Air Force, but after a few months I began to notice the additional loose skin, the lack of pain during an erection, and increased pleasure while masturbating. I began to feel better about myself physically and emotionally. As my restoration has continued (on and off due to deployments) I have reached a better goal than I thought possible at the beginning. My doctors just assume that I am uncircumcised now, guys in the gym or at the nudist beach assume the same, and I couldn't be happier. I still want a longer foreskin with full "hang-over," but my results thus far have made me a happier, more confident man and I love that.

I am still disappointed at my parent's decision to have me circumcised, but I'm not angry with them any more. I know they wanted what they thought was best for me. I've determined never to circumcise any of my children, though. I refuse to put them through what I went through growing up.

Robert
28 years
Texas, USA
11 January 2014

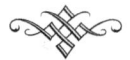

Self-Acceptance

I am an artist who was circumcised at birth because of stupidity and ignorance. I found this was the root of why emotionally I couldn't move past being cut, why it made me feel depressed, and why it was horrible to think about being cut, and why the emotions seemed to often be getting worse instead of better. That's not to say I'm one hundred percent content now and doing everything to restore as fast as possible as if I'm perfect. I still hate being cut and I can still do more to restore. However, I have been getting back into restoration completely effortlessly, which is to say that I do not feel at odds with myself trying to restore. If I'm "shoulding" myself and trying to force restoring, then I make a special effort not to do anything, so I think the fact that I am getting back into restoring says a lot for my emotional state. I do sometimes slip back into feeling absolutely dreadful about everything, but intellectually I understand what it is that causes that feeling.

I didn't like the idea of not being as sensitive as I was born to be, but honestly when I thought of all the times masturbating with my cut dick growing up they are fond memories. I didn't know any better and I enjoyed myself a lot. I know that sex and masturbation has a LOT more to it than just cock stimulation, and I'm very good at enjoying myself and never felt like being cut was a huge barrier. I knew I would much prefer to look uncut, but, as with anything else aesthetic, it only felt really horrible that I didn't look as I felt I should because of deeper issues. There are a million things about myself that I could want to improve physically, but my penis carried the most emotional weight.

I was never personally teased or whatever because of my dick, so I didn't have any of that kind of emotional trauma to move past. But there was *something* really horrible about it all that made me feel really sorry for myself and made the idea of acceptance of being cut overwhelming. I couldn't put my finger on it but I knew it was there and it was so bad that I couldn't even tug (except for the odd moments) for months on end because I was too busy feeling depressed about it and couldn't even find the will to improve my dick physically.

I realized, though, that the heart of it is the feeling that because my dick isn't as good as it could be, then I am not good enough and not worthy enough to be loved. The feeling that my dick made me unworthy of acceptance and love, made me feel ashamed of myself. According to my mind, other people, uncut people, had better dicks and were therefore more worthy of love and acceptance than me. I didn't measure up so, therefore, I am intrinsically worse than them. I would blame my not being good enough on my parents, on society, and I couldn't get over the anger.

Even worse was when after a while of not restoring, it wasn't only something that was done to me, but my dick not having enough skin was MY fault, too. I wasn't good enough and worthy enough and when I had a reason to blame myself for it all, then things got really bad, and I had the hardest time getting back into restoration because of it. I would feel shame for being cut, shame for not being closer to being restored, shame for not putting in the effort.

But the truth is we are all worthy of love, we are good enough. We just need to love ourselves and accept ourselves. Whether or not our penises are cut is just a detail if we learn to love ourselves fully without judgment. We can still enjoy the journey to create our new foreskins and we can still feel that cutting is a terrible thing to force on people. But having circumcision rule our emotions is optional, as long as we know we are worthy of love, regardless of whatever our dick is like.

I'm not entirely where I want to be, but I'm getting there, and by far the biggest thing for me about all of this is learning how important self-love is.

UpwardsLemon
22 years
Canada
21 April 2013

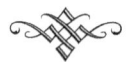

Shame, Guilt, Despair

Shame is such a powerful weapon. Not only is it wrong to question whether circumcision might lead to serious psychological trauma, but it is so wrong that the circumcised man must be shamed and ridiculed as a lesson to others. I have to keep silent about what is most on my mind around family, friends, and professional therapists. Even on foreskin restoration websites, there is a definite split in attitudes about the extent to which circumcision can affect a person's psychology.

I used to think it was my parent's divorce that must have started my severe and chronic social anxiety and depression, but the feelings I have towards that are so mild compared to the sharp downturn in my life from puberty onwards. This, to me, lends more credence to suspecting circumcision as a cause, because I remember all the anguish and anxiety started right during the time that I was awakening sexually.

Maybe it's impossible to get answers. But I sure wish I had one person who I could sit and talk to and explore with, without feeling ashamed and guilty, as if I were the one doing something horrible. I think I resent the silencing more than anything.

I can forgive mistakes, but not when I am the one being continually punished because of the mistakes of others.

I should take it like a man? Why couldn't you wait until I was more than a helpless infant before subjecting me to your blood ritual? What am I supposed to think, as a man, to know I was brutalized in a way that even the worst criminals could not legally be?

Whenever I hear people talk about tolerance, protecting the weak, forgiveness and gratitude, I think of the horror that was inflicted on me that not a soul is sorry for. All those platitudes and ideals just look like empty words. My own words are empty, too. They express little, and do nothing to alleviate my despair.

Brian
30 years
Hawaii, USA
30 November 2013

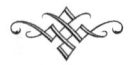

Skin Bridge Removal Diary

Doctor's Appointment - 13 September 2013

A few weeks ago I finally managed to find a doctor who was accepting patients, as I was trying to get my skin bridges removed. After the usual questions about family history and such, she asked me if I had any medical concerns. At first I said "not realllllly" and so she asked again.

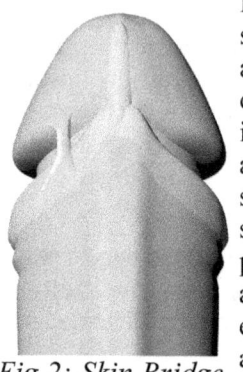

Fig 2: Skin Bridge

I told her it was regarding my penis, and I asked her if she knew what a skin bridge was. She shook her head and said she had no idea what a skin bridge was. (I don't blame her!) So I gave her the quick scoop about improper care/healing, etc., after a circumcision. She asked if I would be willing to allow her to examine me so I said, "Yes, of course." Once I was on the table I showed her what I meant, pointing out each one on my penis. She seemed very sympathetic over the matter and clearly saw my problem. I mentioned the painful erections and the problems that they have caused me and that I was thinking about getting them removed. She said she would refer me to a very good urologist in the city. In the notes she typed up she put my concerns and that it was a "bad circumcision." I guess she didn't fully grasp how skin bridges come about, but no matter.

Urologist's Appointment - 26 September 2013

Right when I walked in the door the urologist was saying goodbye to a patient and after giving my health card to the desk, the doctor saw me in. He quickly asked me the usual questions (smoking, married, etc.) and then asked me to show him the bridges. I dropped my pants and showed him, he nodded and said "Yes, yes these will have to be released," and showed me quickly where the incisions would be made. He said the surgery would be very, very easy, only taking about five minutes and that I would be sore for a day. He said I should get them removed, since as time goes on they have a higher chance of tearing and causing infection.

I proceeded to ask him a few questions. He said there would be no loss of sensitivity in the areas. When asked about scarring and stitches he said its hard to tell until he starts the surgery, but he said that there would probably be minimal scarring, if anything, and that I might get lucky and not need any stitches. It would heal quickly and, as I live in Canada, it would cost me nothing. The only risks would be bleeding and infection.

When asked if he had any experience with skin bridge removals he said, "Yes, I have done many, too many. It's time to quit!" To be double sure, I said, "I DO NOT want another circumcision" and he said, "Of course not. Do not worry. I will only take away the skin that is causing you problems no more, no less." He seemed very knowledgeable and he spoke quickly. I was out of there in three minutes.

I assumed the surgery would involve getting an injection in my penis to numb it, followed with a mild sedative to mellow me out during the operation. The thought of anything sharp poking or cutting my penis makes me nervous. It looks like my penis will have to have surgery two times too many, but I am trying to keep a positive outlook. The bridges would be with me forever; a needle prick will be with me for ten seconds.

Blood Test - 14 October 2013

I went in for a simple blood test in preparation for the surgery. I was cool as a cucumber until the needle came out. I did my best to try to take my mind off it. My heart was still racing and in the end, I was short of breath. I was very nervous—I suppose I have a slight fear of needles.

That was only a tiny little needle in the arm. How the hell am I going to take a needle to my penis? I imagine the vast majority of men out there will never have a needle anywhere near their genital area. I shouldn't say that I could easily have been one of those men if I wasn't circumcised, but that is how I'm feeling at the moment.

Skin Bridge Surgery - 13 November 2013

I was very nervous at the hospital. My girlfriend drove me, and we went to the reception desk to check in. I asked the receptionist what surgery I would be receiving and she said a circumcision (as if I wasn't worried enough). My girlfriend and I told her I was not here for that, but a skin bridge removal. The lady called the operating team and exchanged words. She said it was just a general term and for me not to worry, etc.

Not too convinced, we hopped in the elevator to the surgery floor and met with a nurse. Once again we told her I was not here for a circumcision and asked if I would be able to see the doctor before surgery and she said yes. She told me not to worry as the doctor probably just put it down as a "circ. for x, y and z."

I got into the goofy gown and stayed in a recovery room with my girlfriend. I was extremely nervous as I figured I wouldn't see the doc first, or I would get circumcised again. If it wasn't for my girlfriend being there to support me, there was no way I could have gone through with this. I cannot thank her enough for being so supportive with all of this. She reminded me of the first meeting I had with the doc, which went extremely well. He showed me where he'd cut the bridges and that he wouldn't take off anything else, just the skin that was causing me problems. We must have waited for forty-five minutes and I calmed down much more and wasn't worrying as much.

Another nurse came and took me to the surgery waiting room where he put me on a bed and gave me an IV and explained what was to happen. He showed me the surgical documents for me to sign stating I was to receive a partial frenectomy.[167] Once again I stated the fact that I did not want a full circumcision or anything like that, just the bridges removed. He was a very nice nurse and helped me greatly. The nurse said I would receive the freezing needle in my penis first before I was to be sedated, which worried me as I knew I would be one hundred percent awake for it. The anesthetist visited me and we discussed the options and decided on the penis needle and sedation. He said I would not remember much of the surgery, and I would wake up after and be okay.

The urologist swung by next and told me not to worry—he wasn't going to circumcise me; he would only remove the lesions. At this point I was sure I would not have to worry about being accidentally circumcised again. I started to build up my courage, as the needle would be arriving soon. I was taken into the operation room where the anesthetist began hooking me up to a machine to measure my heart rate, etc. I stated one more time to the team I did not want a circumcision, just the skin bridges.

I also stated I had not received the freezing yet either as I was supposed to get it in the recovery room. The anesthetist told me he was going to administer the sedative drugs now as he felt it would be better for me not having to have a needle down there. The nurses were all very kind and the anesthetist was very nice. He placed the drug into my IV and gave me some oxygen. Next thing I knew I was awake in the recovery room a little sleepy.

After I woke up more I was taken back to my beautiful girlfriend, who I was very happy to see. I got dressed, had a small snack and some juice, and we were on our way home (not before stopping to pick up some prescriptions for me).

The bandage on my penis is very clean and secure. I am to remove it by soaking it in water in two days. Apart from taking antibiotics, T3's and

---

[167] *Frenectomy* is the surgical removal of the frenulum.

making sure I am looking after the wounds, I should be back to normal in two to three weeks. I am anxious and nervous to take off the bandages but I must wait as I do not want to mess anything up. I have no pain on my penis, except for a very tiny sensation I can feel on the underside of my penis. There is a tiny bit of swelling near my urethra that causes some discomfort rubbing against my underwear. So far no giant pain, no blood, and I've made it through an erection or two with no trouble as of yet. From what I can tell, I was not circumcised as the top of my glans and shaft feel completely normal, which makes me very relieved.

The only thing that has got me a little bit worried is that the papers said partial frenectomy. Not that I have a frenulum anymore to remove, mind you. It's very hard to pinpoint where the sensation is coming from on my penis, especially with it all bandaged up. So it would do me no good to worry. He said he would remove the bridges and that's it. There were no bridges close to my "frenulum area" so it would have been pointless to cut there again. If you think about it a frenulum is similar to a skin bridge in certain aspects, i.e. it being connected to the glans. I doubt there is a fancy medical word for removing a skin bridge so the frenectomy term was used. Most people don't even know what a skin bridge is, so with that knowledge I am feeling better now. The doc didn't see me after, as he had more patients, so I can assume everything went as planned.

Post-Surgery - 15 November 2013

Once again I woke up with no blood/pain/anything. My penis still feels like it always has except for the bandages and slight swelling with the urethra again. I've been taking the antibiotics on time, as well as painkillers when needed (haven't taken any except for the first day as a precaution).

After my beautiful girlfriend brought me lunch, we proceeded to the bathroom to begin removing the bandages. We soaked my penis in the salt water for a minute, then slowly began to remove the medical tape. After the tape was mostly off, we soaked again. The bandage was coming off fairly easily as we took off the layers. We finally got to the last layer and I was very nervous to see what was done. The top of my penis had been left alone, as I had thought. My girlfriend took the first look and told me only the bridges had been touched. Relieved, we soaked my penis one last time and carefully removed the last bandage. Removing everything didn't hurt at all. My penis is a little swollen and looks pretty funny from the slight ballooning in the area where the bridges had been cauterized—three spots on the bottom of my glans, and four spots on my shaft where the bridges used to be. Whew! Talk about a sigh of relief! I quickly had a shower, being careful of my penis, and we wrapped it back up, putting a small amount of Vaseline on the wounds, then a sterile pad followed by wrapping it in a bandage with tape.

The journey is almost over, and now I just have to heal. I can't thank my amazing girlfriend enough for everything she's done for me.

Young Man
22 years
Canada
September–November 2013

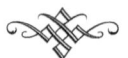

Subconscious Damage And Hypocrisy

I accepted my circumcision and, growing up, was brain-washed into believing it was better to be circumcised as it was "cleaner." I felt "superior" to the other boys at school who had been left uncut and at that time it was incomprehensible to me that one of my intact friends, whose mother was a medical doctor, had left him intact. Didn't she know?

It always bothered me that I looked so unhappy in the family album photographs. During childhood and growing up I was always "adjusting" (making myself comfortable by pulling my foreskin remnant over my glans). In fact this became a bit of a "joke" with my sisters—that my hand was forever in my pants! At the beginning of every new school semester there would appear in the newspaper an advert for boys' underwear which said "send him back to school in comfort." On reflection, the foreskin is the most comfortable covering for the penis.

So why was I so unhappy in the family photographs? I had a loving family upbringing. Two parents, a brother and two sisters. We were all well and healthy. I realize that subconsciously I was living in the fear of being fully castrated.—After all, if my parents, who were supposed to protect me, had allowed me to be circumcised, couldn't they allow further damage?

One school holiday, my mother returned from the shops visibly shaken. I was home and must have been about twelve. Before starting her family she had been a nursery school teacher (and so loved children). What had upset her was that in the shop she had overheard a mother saying to her little boy, "If you don't behave, I will cut it off."

She was shocked that someone could say this to a child, as children take things in a literal manner. She understood the mother to mean "I will cut your penis off." But I thought it somewhat hypocritical (unintended) of my mother as she had allowed the doctors to cut off my foreskin (part of my penis).

My mother had one brother and four sisters. Her brother was intact, as was her father. Sadly, she married my father, who was circumcised, and so the decision to have my brother and I circumcised was left to him. Perhaps, if my mother had been more aware of the functions of the foreskin, she may not have married my father or allowed us to be sexually mutilated.

I am trying to restore the protective and linear bearing[168] that the foreskin is. There are many unique bits, the frenulum and frenular (ridged) band, that I will not be able to repair. They are gone for good. Very sad.

Parents should realize that in having their sons circumcised they are condemning their future daughters-in-law to a lifetime of frustrating and painful sex.

Why are we so arrogant that we feel that we can improve on God's or Evolution's design? Every other male mammal species has a foreskin. Clearly it is there for a reason. So amputating it is pure ignorance.

Georged
53 years
South Africa
6 November 2013

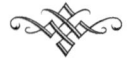

---

[168] The foreskin acts as a linear bearing because it provides for free movement back and forth.

Swallowing The Red Pill

I'm a Caucasian male. I was circumcised on the fourth day after my birth, but I never really knew what that meant. It was entirely absent from my high school biology/anatomy and sex education classes. I never really thought about it.

I'm at college now, and only about two months ago did I really look at my scar on my penis and question what happened. So I looked it up, and read. Read a lot: an awful, awful, horrific, heart-eviscerating lot. I asked two of my best friends if they had ever realized and thought about what happened. They most certainly had. And they were fucking pissed just like me.

Worse yet, one is a medical student, and the other is a biomedical engineer. Both mentioned how the human prepuce had been notably absent or vaguely described in their textbooks. And this wasn't just anywhere, some random ass medical school. This was goddamn Johns Hopkins Medical University, one of the top, if not the top, medical schools in the country.

At that point, I hadn't read about the nerves in the ridged band or the preputial sphincter [foreskin opening] or the mucosa that acts as an emollient for the glans. I just knew that something was missing. So I did more reading. I consumed everything.

I felt as though the freedom and all pervasive knowledge of the Internet was Morpheus, and he had presented me with the Blue Pill and the Red Pill. [169] As all circumcised men who are able to completely off rip the blinders that society imposes through lies of omission know, the latter is a hard one to swallow.

I have always had an amputation fear. I knew that if I ever lost an arm, or a leg, that I probably would prefer death to living without a whole human body. I realized, when I figuratively swallowed the red pill that I was indeed an amputee, and had been all my life except for three days.

Over the past three weeks I have cried enough to leave myself constantly dehydrated. I tried to talk to my parents, but as soon as I said I was angry about being circumcised, they instantly dismissed me. I felt abandoned by the only people that I should always feel I could turn to. My mother, life

---

[169] To the Ancient Greeks, Morpheus was the leader of the spirits of dreams and provided a deceptive reality to sleepers. In the film *The Matrix*, Neo has the choice of a blue pill that would allow him to remain in the fabricated world of the matrix (as most circumcised men remain in a 'coma') or the red pill that would allow him to escape and enter reality.

herself, refused to cradle and comfort me like the baby she always considers me. My father, a Jewish man who eats bacon and never goes to temple, gave the answer, "I was Jewish, it's tradition, something I pass on to you." That's all he had to say.

I'll pass on the details, but my mother and father said they "knew" it was just a piece of skin, that I was making such a huge deal out of nothing, and even threatened to disown me ("It's your father's religion! You need to think about [it] if you want to continue to be a member of this family!"). They absolutely refused to even talk about it, much less view any information I had that shows what a barbaric, ritualistic, partial dick amputation it really is.

As far as most people I know, parents included, they think the foreskin is just extra penile shaft skin. Cut a little off, there's still everything else left. My father never questioned it his whole life; he couldn't understand why I was/am. To make the pain even worse, he revealed to me that my grandfather is intact. I don't know how my grandfather, having lived his life with a working, sensual dick, could circumcise his son, even if he was Jewish!

I have to vent this out, too. My mother is Methodist, and again, not devout. She never goes to church, or does anything remotely religious. When I was born they agreed not to force any religion on my mind and let me grow and decide on my own. That was nice of them. Too bad they let my dad impose his religion on my body instead.

I only found solace and people who would listen to me in the form of my dog, my girlfriend, and my cousin (also Jewish-born, but not Jewish himself ... still circumcised though).

Suicide and the reckless hunting of my circumciser (who is alive, and I happen to have his name, his picture, addresses) have crossed my mind. I realize that's part of the grieving process. In the past few days I've been able to function, but I still have that ever-present emotional ache and dread in the back of my mind every day. I'm probably correct in the assumption that it never goes away.

I've heard horror stories from men who can't get it up by age forty or fifty. These are the men who barely feel anything and pound their wives into ground beef in order to orgasm and who go through five tubes of lube a month just to chafe their wife to death. I figure making a substitute foreskin can help with a lot of that.

It really hit me hard as a brick when I read about all the parts removed. It even made perfect sense. I'm "lucky" enough to have my frenulum still, and I have enough slack skin when flaccid to cover 80% of my glans if I pull it forward at that moment. The only way I can orgasm is with a lot of handgrip pressure, and I realized I always put an index finger where it can rub the frenulum—if I don't, I can't orgasm. How fucked up is that? Makes perfect sense. Plus, like everyone else, my glans is dry and cracked and barely feels a thing besides pain.

My girlfriend tried using her mouth on me for a while and I was so underwhelmed—I could barely feel a thing. Granted, she had zero experience, so she wasn't doing much besides licking a lollipop, but I was so depressed because I couldn't feel the tactile surface of her tongue or the warmth of her mouth. I thought it was some cruel joke of nature that my fingertips could feel her more than my dick could.

It all makes such perfect, horrible, outrageous sense now.

I feel as though my life will never be what it could have been. Fifteen minutes of surgery, and a lifetime of deprivation, shame, psychological trauma, and wondering "what if?"

And the bastard is still alive.

On the more constructive side, I've decided to start restoring. I'm slack enough when flaccid as is, why the fuck not, right? Surprisingly enough, even my girlfriend, who is a Muslim, supports me. Granted, she doesn't understand it, but she knows and has seen my pain.

Thanks for reading all that, if you did. It's a freaking essay. Maybe my parents can read it one day.

Jeffrey
25 years
Manhattan, USA
21 April 2010

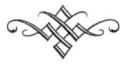

Talking With My Parents

I just finished a long talk with my parents about how I feel about circumcision. I told them how I see it as mutilation and how I see it as disgustingly unfair that women are protected and men are not. I even showed them a list of what is lost from circumcision and what could go wrong. My father kept saying, "Look, it says here 'has not been studied in depth'" every time it came up, like it was an excuse.

I told them how I feel like half of a man—that I feel incomplete. I told them that what they had done to me has ruined my life, whether they had thought they were doing the right thing at the time or not.

My father said that all of the uncut men he has ever known had infections. I know this is not true. How do I reply to this? My mother said she thought the foreskin was gross. I told her "you think a dried out cut up penis is better?" All I want them to do is to look me in the eyes and tell me they are genuinely sorry they had me circumcised, and sorry about how it has affected me.

I even told them that I have been restoring for a year and a half. I said, "It's like I'm slowly molding a black and white TV to a fairly decent color TV, but it still makes me angry knowing I'm supposed to have an HD TV with surround sound and 1000 channels in the first place."

Joseph
23 years
Oregon, USA
19 October 2011

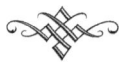

The Eternal Scream

I have thought about how to express my anger at having my penis mutilated as a newborn infant. I wish to explain the various ways this has truly been an eternal scream for me, something that has affected all aspects of my life.

Truthfully, the best way is really to watch one of these operations and hear the screams of the poor child. I don't like to use that poor child as a guinea pig, but his suffering might as well cause some good in the world.

Many of the things I am going to say I never knew why I thought them or did them until recently. As a toddler, I tried to no avail to shove my penis head back into the foreskin. The reason was because it felt more comfortable and was less irritating to me when it was shoved into the foreskin. Granted, I couldn't get it to hold there without some effort and I eventually gave up, but I did try.

As I grew and became a teenager I was always struck by the fact I thought my penis looked odd. I always thought it looked wrong or even sick. My penis, however, looked like every other penis I had seen—except for one guy's I saw that was seemingly just about shoved all the way into his balls. It looked small and had a huge pee hole. When I discovered circumcision and its horrible effects and saw pictures of circumcised penises gone exceptionally wrong, one looked exactly like this penis I remember seeing. Poor fellow, it is a shame my teenage self didn't know that's why his penis looked something out of a sci-fi movie experiment.

As I became a young adult, and even as an adult, my penis always looked sick to me. It never looked healthy, but I couldn't figure out why. So, I've always thought my penis looked wrong, but I never knew why this was the case. Perhaps this is why I am pee shy? Perhaps it is because I am at my deepest levels ashamed of my own naked body because I see it as deformed?

Throughout a large chunk of my life I would say I have had a recurring nightmare/dream/daydream of sorts. For some reason I kept having a repeated nightmare of my penis getting cutting off. I didn't know what the area that kept getting cut off was called, like I do now. Apparently for a large chunk of my life I've had a dream about my penis getting cut off right around the mutilation scar. Very rarely was this nightmare cutting off any other area of my penis. I can't forget it. It's always either a knife or scissors going down there in a dark room and hacking it off, and I'm defenseless, yet not tied down and screaming in agony. It has been a lifelong agonizing nightmare. Yes, I have gotten used to it, but I truly wonder if it isn't connected to my mutilation. I wonder if my infant cries for help that went unheeded have caused me to dream about my penis getting cut off right around my circumcision scar for the past 30 years? When I first had this dream I screamed and it was terrifying, but it never went away. I now cry, knowing I am just reliving over and over and over again something that happened from during my first hours of life.

I've also learned that the chronic random pain my penis experiences is from my scar to where the penis head starts. This pain is especially apparent after I have masturbated. Not every single time, but enough that I've noticed.

I've learned my lost foreskin would make it easier to masturbate without porn. Is this a cause of my porn addiction? Furthermore, porn doesn't help in getting women—it actually makes it worse. Is this, plus the fact I have a mutilated penis, plus I've always thought my penis looked sick and kept dreaming of it getting cut off, another reason I suck with women?

I was born with the umbilical cord strangling me. Perhaps my infant self had wanted to die before being mutilated. This might sound crazy, but babies in the womb do hear things. I was, however, revived because I was born lifeless. This was a trauma, a fact I know simply because it damaged my nerves in my ears giving me a hearing impairment and who knows what else. The doctors called it birth trauma. I am not mad about this as they succeeded in reviving me. But, I cannot help but wonder what effect that had on me along with the trauma of having my penis mutilated shortly thereafter. I imagine it takes a cruel sick monster to revive a dead baby only to mutilate his genitals while telling the poor baby it is for his own good.

I know growing up I had a natural distrust of women. I never bonded with my parents, especially my mother. As a teenager the relationship between my mom and me got even more strained, to the point where something occurred and I forgot two years of my life. As time went on, I did eventually forgive her in my heart. I never told her because every time I looked at the issue and thought about it there was some unspeakable thing I couldn't place my fingers on that I couldn't forgive. I thought on it and soul searched and really tried to come to peace with it. I thought I had, but then I stumbled onto circumcision.

As a teenager I suffered much depression and suicidal tendencies. I became a bit fixated on the darker elements of life. I have to wonder how much of this is a result of my birth traumas. I cannot say 100% one way or the other but I am willing to say with 90% certainty that much of the pain I've described is a result of my infancy and its trauma—my double birth trauma. I read much about the topic.

I even partly understood it and wasn't completely mad, but then I watched a circumcision video. I first saw a link to one and it took me two days of thinking before I decided to click on it and watch it. I was horrified. It was like an old memory hit me and it hit me hard. I normally do not become emotionally unglued, but I couldn't stop screaming at the computer. I cried for many hours. I truly was wroth with anger.

I was overcome with a desire to torture these monsters. They need to be castrated without anesthetics (with smelling salts on hand so they can be woken up in case they pass out) and the old fashioned way with scissors and then locked in jail. They need to have mirrors placed in positions where they can see the operation, and tape placed on their eyes lest they shut their eyes and don't watch. These people need to suffer. I'd be all for doing human experimentation on these "doctors." One good start might be repeating the crimes in the movie *Human Centipede*. My point is that they need to suffer, and I need to hear them scream, preferably while, like the babies, being told how this is for their own good.

You know, while watching a circumcision video, it really was like I remembered my own. I seem to recall a terrible pain and scream. I know my infant self was doing nothing short of vowing to get revenge. It might seem too strange to have a newborn memory, but it really truly is like recovering a lost memory and finding out the lost memory was of a time you were raped. I know in what I've written I haven't come across as too angry aside from one paragraph, but my anger is beyond words. There are no words for my anger, so I did not bother expressing it at every turn, so instead I wanted to explain how this has affected my life.

My vision of seeing a newborn baby boy getting his penis mutilated is like watching a terrible nightmare. It is like watching a real life horror movie. I imagine the poor child first screaming and no one cares. As his penis is set up I see the Devil beginning to laugh. As his penis is poked at, I can hear the frantic laughter of hell around him and I can see the chain of the bond with his mother being nearly broken. I can see the devils' chains that drag a soul to hell grabbing this poor child as the "good" doctor does the bidding of all that is evil. As the majority of the foreskin is cut I hear the most horrific scream being let out—a scream that reaches throughout the entire universe. I see the heavens weeping at the gift of free will that man does have. I see tears coming from God and the angels. As the last bit of foreskin is ripped apart, as the doctor always needs to get a little straggling foreskin, the baby cries one last time and in this instance this pure and innocent child is blackened.

His bond with Mom is broken and is replaced with the Devil's chain which is now the bond he will have with Mom. His guardian angel, known as "Mom," has now become his guardian devil. I see throughout this the eternal scream that from that moment on will follow the child for his entire life. This scream will ensure his sex life is bad, his penis will be deformed, his brain will be altered, his manhood will be destroyed, and a whole host of other things will follow him, making this his very eternal never ending scream. Long after his cry pierces the heavens he will carry with him a reminder that humanity is a wicked and vile creation. He will be reminded that God did weep and repent for making His creation known as Man during the days of Noah's flood. The Devil will continue living in the house and bodies of doctors who perform these surgeries. This boy will forever know that mankind uses its gift of free will for pure uncensored, unadulterated evil.

You can learn much about a society by how it treats its children. I am an American and I truly love the ideals and the constitution and what our founders created. I am a Christian and I truly do love the gospel principles, but for this I can have no forgiveness. A quick note for Christians and Mormon Christians: your scriptures do condemn this act. The New Testament says it is like believing there is no Christ and, Mormons, your scriptures call it Solemn Mockery of God. You, my fellow Christians, do solemnly mock the same God you claim to worship.

The cries of these baby boys in America do damn us all. The fact we don't do it to baby girls also tells me baby boys are of little value. America has turned into a society of women that damns the men. The leader of the world, the lone super power has said if you are a boy you are evil. What hope is there for this country when the screams of baby boys do damn us before a just God? I am saddened. I am angry and I do weep for it all. May God have mercy on our souls for what we have done with the privileges that come with living in a country that is the leader of the free world.

How can the next generation of men grow up to be men when they are really half-men whose very manhood has been damn near amputated? They are almost neutered. What manner of men are these then? I weep for myself and America for "castrating" its newborn baby boys. My cries are loud and they are endless. If my possible future sons can hear me, I will have to be killed before I let them "castrate" you. God, send me your sons: they will be safe in my hands. That is the only silver lining for me.

Kayne
29 years
South Carolina, USA
28 February 2014

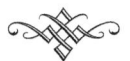

The Gardener

Again, the razor
Has kissed my lips,
Lapping sweetly
At the dew which drips.

He hungers the flavor,
He harbors no regrets,
He covets the membranes he gets.

The altar is set,
Ritual begins
No trauma yet
Quivering violet,
How your bud glistens.
Gardener violent,
Shearing is part of
The system. Shrill,
Shrill are the shrieks as he snips him!

Grill of nails, mad man,
Gnashing down upon
The stem. Blue rose,
Your petals are peeled,
Raw and exposed!

The Gardener

Skinned alive, unnatural
Retracted are the jaws
Sinews sticky he licks
Gulping down the petals.
Rosebud writhing, screaming
In horror as he rips.

Pale young flower,
Once vibrant, now dreadfully sick!
Earth bloodied with milky leaf tips.

The razor has shorn the blossom,
Destroying the pollen.
Sensorial lamina flayed,
The vibrant vine has fallen.
Bud badly mutilated—
Forlorn, Forever.

Jaime Banks
30 years
Pennsylvania, USA
31 December 2013

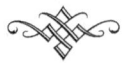

The Journey To My Real Manhood

When I look back at the voyage of my life,
Sometimes, I just want to cry,
I'm missing something, not knowing what,
When I'm just being myself, I'm ashamed, too shy,
I walk around questioning this inner beast,
What could I be missing? I scream aloud,
Receiving only silence, no answers,
Just stares all around.

I never gave the bond between nature and man a thought,
Until I discovered what happened to me,
A sacrifice, unnecessary, cruel, barbaric,
The reason for my incompleteness, a kind of slavery,
Every day I realize, is like an anniversary of sadness,
Thinking about the burden on my soul,
The cut being deeper than they thought, scarring my heart,
For what I would not give to be once again whole.

Trying to cope, searching the world over, I think I've found a way,
I've made my decision and I'm restoring the pieces of me,
Though I may never be whole again, I must think to never give in,
In hopes to strike a balance with harmony,
There may be hardships along the road,
Criticism, impatience, and being cast aside,
But though far off, peace of mind is still in range,
I must remember this is a journey to my real manhood,
The true life I'm creating with the turning of every page.

The Journey To My Real Manhood

The pain I've endured,
Knowing the suffering of my plight,
Of being violated, robbed, desecrated,
This is why I as well as many other men fight,
Going to the battlefield,
To assure that no other boy might,
Lose this most precious part,
The foreskin, his God-given, natural birthright.

One day after I'm gone,
I pray deeply for the world to open its eyes,
So that it will stop this torture, this inhumanity,
As no man should live his life in lies,
Trying to stay strong, hold together, that he really is normal,
Because after all, he was given no choice,
To remain beautiful, intact, healthy, and natural,
The circumcisions must stop
And when that day happens every male will rejoice.

Kohiro Hakuya
Georgia, USA
21 years
2009

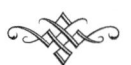

The Power Of Restoring

My mother hadn't really planned on having me cut and really wasn't sure it was a good idea in the first place. My dad never gave it a second thought because at the time I was born (1971), the father wasn't allowed anywhere near the delivery area. My father was cut as an infant as well (rare in 1937) and he really had no opinion on the matter.

My mother ended up being convinced by the obstetrician who said: "It's vestigial and not needed. It's good hygiene and the procedure is very, very quick—only a minute or two. It won't hurt for very long." He was the best obstetrician in the city, supposedly, and my mother figured he knew what was best. He convinced her, and though she didn't see the procedure, she was in the same room when it was done.

She said I screamed and it upset her, but she really thought it would be in my best interest and she thought a moment of pain I wouldn't remember was worth a lifetime of good hygiene. She said the doctor was true to his word and I only cried for a minute or two and it never bothered me again. Who knows if that meant it was indeed quick or I went into shock. I'll never know and she won't either.

I never gave it a second thought until I saw one performed. I almost vomited. I don't remember ever reacting to anything as strongly as I did to that sight.

My revulsion turned to fury. I felt utterly betrayed and like I had been branded as either a Jew (which I wasn't) or an American (which, of course, I am). I was seething with rage. Fortunately, I discovered foreskin restoration at the time I was researching. That was my answer and restoring my foreskin would be the great big "fuck you" to the medical establishment, the doctor, the US, and my mother. I didn't restore for the sensation gains—I had no idea of those at the time—realizing that came later.

I have to remember this was 1971, when everyone was basically clueless and doctors were God's personal assistants. It took me a long, long time to forgive my parents—a decade almost. It wasn't enough to affect our relationship, which is quite good, but it was resentment in the back of my mind.

It really helped to be able to talk to my parents about it and finally hear the whole story—and understand that they were convinced to do it after being sold a steaming pile of shit disguised as medicine. I can't blame my parents or resent their decision, as they really thought they were doing a good thing and they listened to the doctor, as there was no other choice. I've forgiven them. They now know I am restoring my foreskin, that I'm within a year of getting back all the skin stolen from me, and they both are completely supportive of my restoration.

I started restoring because I was really pissed off, and I realized I could do something about it. I was amazed that I could take my power back. I had no idea what an amazing journey (though not always easy) this would be. It's physically, mentally, and emotionally demanding. It really is. It's not a matter of strapping on a device and waiting a few months. It's an ongoing, dedicated, almost obsessive effort that can take five or more years to complete.

However, the rewards are far beyond what I ever suspected they would be when I started. It's beyond edifying. The first time someone else thought I was intact it was all worth it! Though it's a hassle and a definite long-term commitment to yourself, it's very empowering—you never, ever take your foreskin for granted and you have a sense of personal accomplishment and pride that no intact man will ever have.

I restored from 1999-2001, reaching a Coverage Index (CI) of 5. I started up again in 2005 for about six months, reaching a CI-6. I was content with that until last summer. I've been restoring again since July 2012 and I'm a CI-8 now in late 2013. I want to reach a CI-9 with 50% erect coverage. By the time I reach that goal I will have been restoring for a total of five years.

This quote below is what got me restoring for the first time in 1999. I don't recall exactly where I read it, but it was on one of the early restoring sites. It has been and still is my overarching goal: *"If you do it right, your restoration will produce a penis that is so similar in appearance and function to an intact one that only your urologist, if he's paying attention, will notice the difference."*

Ian
41 years
Florida, USA
27 October 2013

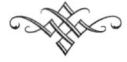

The Procedure—A Short Story

I stand here in the operating room, my head reeling.[170] I've done this many times before: Betadine, Circumstraint, clamp, scalpel, sutures just in case; the cold, steel tray holds all the tools we need. As a nurse in this large public hospital, I am always honored when Dr. Knox asks me to help him. Dr. Knox seems so confident, he loves his work. I respect him. But sometimes I'm not so sure …

Dr. Knox enters the operating room. He's grinning. He lathers up, rinses, lathers again. After all, he wouldn't want any pathogens creeping into the circumcision wound. That's Dr. Knox for you, always thinking of the children. He's a man of average stature, fair hair and sunny disposition. His own kids call him "Dr. Smiley." He's always smiling. That's Dr. Knox for you, ever cheerful. He knows the result he wants: high and tight, clean and dry. The Jews would agree; *brit milah* is a sacred covenant. A child's body, after all, is the canvas upon which we paint our wishes. A hygienic entity is one step from God. The doctor gets it. Besides, tradition illustrates that an act of solidarity is always beneficial.

I once had a coworker, one who did not work in pediatrics, who expressed to me the most curious opinion. She said: "A purloined prepuce is ecstasy wasted and the potential for bodily integrity discarded." She seemed a disturbed individual. Imagine, a grown woman so concerned about a baby boy's genitals. There's something creepy about that. Good thing she prefers cardiology.

The Jews know that the flesh of a man is the sweet ambrosia we offer in ceremony to God. The Muslims get it too. A knife to the flesh, the excision of sensation; that is the way of the healthy. This child is Christian, but he's also American. He has assaulted the world in several ways. First, he was conceived by filthy copulation. Second, he contains the tools of sexual depravity. Third, well, he's male. In America the masses appreciate the allure of perfect symmetry. No religious excuse necessary. Today it is a medical procedure. Hygiene and science are all the dogma we need. Certainly symmetry is not guaranteed, but an effort for perfection pleases the Lord. Sometimes evolution makes mistakes. The foreskin is one example.

---

[170] Although this fictional short story is full of irony, it is an accurate observation of a hidden aspect of American medical culture.

When the doctor carries the pink succulent in like a sacrificial lamb, the babe with translucent skin seems a perfect offering. He says he prefers using soft cotton restraints; Dr. Knox is a warm heart. This little fella's named Henry. His mother asked for low and loose, but we know what Dr. Knox prefers. While analyzing Henry, the doctor decides the incision point. Now he is omnipotent, the infant can offer no caveat. The action of immediate concern is that of tearing the prepuce from the glans. There exists a synechium, a connecting tissue.[171] This penis is sealed shut like a rose bud. The doctor grasps the tip of the foreskin and yanks it back, it tears like a fingernail. First mission accomplished. The infant becomes rigid and emits the most piercing scream I've ever heard; that's saying a lot in my line of work.

I want with all my being to snatch him up and run. But I have a career to think of.

The tender pulp of Henry's inner penis is exposed. It's oozing blood and other secretions. Dr. Knox grasps the penis, brings the clamp down and lays it upon the bleeding glans. The frigid sting of the steel causes the infant's eyes to widen and he releases another shriek. The doctor, his eyes glassy with necessity, screws the clamp tight. He's crushing the tissue with thousands of pounds of pressure; this way death is usually prevented. An occasional hemorrhage resulting in death will be listed as simply that: Cause of Death: Hemorrhage.

Upon application of the scalpel, the skin slides off, a piece of sushi. Only gurgles now emit from the orifice which minutes ago trumpeted a piercing protest. Catatonia is the soundest sleep of all.

The doctor instructs me not to discard the foreskin, for it can be used to help others. The skin will expand in a laboratory and be grafted onto burn victims and other unfortunates. I comply; the prepuce is ushered away by another nurse. The pink baby body is now an intense fuchsia. The indigo veins are quite visible through the translucent skin; he looks like a perfect dumpling.

And like a breathing hunk of ham, he may be flesh and blood, but his body is not his own. "As sentient beings we have the right to rule, we can sculpt our children into anything we want. And if they dare complain, remind them, if it were not for you, they'd have never been born." That's what Dr. Knox tells parents as he presents to them the consent forms.

Sometimes I wonder if The Procedure is ethical. It has been said that the prepuce is the center of male sexual sensation—Meissner's corpuscles

---

[171] The *synechium* is the shared membrane connecting the glans to the inside of the foreskin in young boys.

enervate the triangle of mucosa named the frenular delta. I myself have learned to follow rationality: fine touch is overrated. Besides, Dr. Knox wouldn't steer us wrong, how in the world could he sleep? No, everything is all right. When I ponder how a procedure that removes sexual parts from a neonate could possibly be so benign, let alone beneficial, I remember a conversation I had with the doctor's associate, Dr. Fisher.

Dr. Fisher told me about a friend of his who lost two fingers in a gardening accident as a child. The limbs were gone: nerves, veins, skin ... all were severed and lost. But he experienced the most remarkable phenomenon; he could still feel the fingers! Indeed, he now calls them his "Lil' Phantom Twins." Why, he claimed he could even use them! That's life for you, always presenting miracles. He said, in fact, a three-fingered hand is more efficient than one with five. Phantom fingers are quite agile. And of course, now that he is missing those fingers, his chances of suffering from a hangnail or fracture are substantially reduced. Due to this information, Dr. Fisher recently gathered the resolve, and had amputated the ring and pinkie fingers from his right hand! Now he is just like his friend. He told me he wished he'd had them removed long ago. It makes perfect sense.

I fear I've been off topic again, assuaging the cloying fears which drag me down, the bane of many, I am sure. What's intuition when perception is better served by the intellect of others? My mother always said, "If I say the sky is green and you can see that it is blue, it's green." She was a wise woman. I decided on the green sky long ago. Every time I express any of my doubts, I am surrounded by an array of blinding smiles. They have a talent for coercion, those bright white teeth and twinkling eyes.

Dr. Knox is in the process of removing the clamp at this very moment. The tiny baby's organ is a delicate tulip in full bloom, only with most of its petals removed. The infant's eyes are half-mast, he looks most mild now; the tranquility of surrender attends to him like cherubim. The doctor looks on, still smiling. He tilts his head and sighs. Another job well done; not an increment of glans caught in the melee this time. Not a peep from me, the doctor's complicit subordinate. No, I simply look on and sigh as well.

Mother always said, "The meek shall inherit the Earth." I'm still waiting, I don't know. Sometimes I'm not so sure.

Jaime Banks
30 years
Pennsylvania, USA
31 December 2013

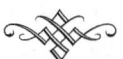

There Are None So Blind...

As a two day old neonate, I was strapped into a Circumstraint to have my genitals mutilated. This was done by and at the insistence of a doctor. He used me as a thing, a means to his own ends, whatever they may have been.

In time, I came to resent what was done without my consent. I restored my foreskin via non-surgical tissue expansion and thus gained first hand experience of what was taken from me. Although it's a long process, there was a dramatic tipping point when the prepuce began to roll over and consistently cover my glans. At this point I noticed a big improvement in my sex life. The hypothetical had become the actual—*and I went crazy*. I did more and more research, and the more I learned, and the more I thought about the ethics involved, the crazier I became. I sought treatment at the Bay Pines Veterans Administration Medical Center, where I was treated by Doctors W and X and Mr. Y.

SENSITIVE AND CONFIDENTIAL DOCUMENT
DATE/TIME: 29 MAY 2013 @ 1005
PATIENT RELATES UNUSUAL BELIEF THAT HIS CIRCUMSISION[SIC] AT AGE OF 2 DAYS WAS IN AND OF ITSELF A "RAPE" ... CONSIDER[S] CIRCUMCISION TO HAVE BEEN "MUTILATING"...
SIGNED BY: DR W

Dr W. stated a number of times that "The last thing we want to do is make things worse." However, the more they treated me, the worse I felt—the rage would wash over me like a wave that left me dizzy. From the beginning they wrote about my feelings in sneer quotes. It became clear that they had the same approach to medicine as my assailant when they started making decisions without consulting me.

SENSITIVE AND CONFIDENTIAL DOCUMENT
06/17/2013 ADDENDUM STATUS: COMPLETED
PATIENT'S RECORDS WERE REVIEWED AND CASE WAS DISCUSSED WITH DR. W. PATIENT DOES NOT SEEM APPROPRIATE FOR GROUP THERAPY
SIGNED: DR W, 06/17/2013 16:54; DR X, 06/18/2013 08:43

Dr. W wanted me to have Cognitive Behavioral Therapy, and I asked about evenings and weekends to avoid missing time at work. They had a meeting which I was not present for and decided without my approval to transfer me to Dr. X. They did not consider the impact on my finances, nor did they consider the transference problem that I warned of; Dr. X is also a victim of genital mutilation. When Mr Y phoned me to inform me of the change, he blatantly lied to me, saying that "Dr. Z is not available, so we need to reschedule you ... ." He would later write that I was "paranoid" because I complained about his lie—*which is clearly documented in my medical records.*

I ALSO OFFERED HIM THERAPY THAT MIGHT EASE THE EMOTIONAL IMPACT OF HIS KNOWLEDGE OF HIS CIRCUMCISION, BY HELPING HIM TO ACCEPT WHAT HAD HAPPENED IN THIS REGARD, BUT HE WAS NOT INTERESTED. Dr X.

Knowing nothing of circumcision, Dr. X wrote of my "apparent obsession with ... having been circumcized [sic] as an infant ... (which he considers 'rape') ..." and of my trying to engage him in philosophical discussions. He rationalized my pain away as a political issue, likening me to pro-lifers. It never occurred to him that not a single pro-lifer is an aborted fetus. It never occurred to him that I had been sexually assaulted—and his task was to treat that. I asked him if I *had been* sexually assaulted, or if I *felt as though I were.* Showing zero insight he presented a series of rationalizations, such as I don't remember, I don't know the difference, et cetera. When I pressed him he admitted that they were all invalid—but not that it is a sexual assault. He blamed me for his own failure to provide meaningful treatment.

The next time I saw Dr. W, he also said that this is a political issue. This was their plan. They would insist that I speak about my self-esteem, and stop wasting their time with this "political issue." They would decide what is best for me. They would gang up on me and force their plans on me. *It never occurred to them that I was there because a doctor had done that to me.* This amplified my rage and directed it at them. As my self-esteem had improved I decided that I was no longer going to put up with this. I decided that our relationship was over.

Dear Dr. W,
"I am sorry that you are feeling it hard to connect with me and Dr. X."
An odd statement, as connecting with patients is contrary to your treatment philosophy.
"We find often-times that this ... can actually serve as a point to help in your progress if you can try to work ... through your concerns with me and Dr. X."
I'm not sanguine that my loss of patience heralds the change which is required in you.
Cheers,
~Thomas

However, it's not so simple. Dr. W. would have to agree to let me see someone else—and they had already decided to force themselves on me. The definition of incompetence is a failure to understand the limits of one's abilities; thus a person cannot be the judge of his own competence. I refused to see him, and sent a string of secure messages telling him how much I hated him. Being completely clueless, he thought that we were on the verge of a breakthrough, and kept saying that we should work through this. He was overconfident in his abilities—to the point of delusion.

In the end I walked into the emergency room and spoke to the psychiatrist on duty. She felt that I needed to be on medication and offered to commit me voluntarily. She then remembered that Dr W. happened to be on vacation and told me to go as a walk-in the next morning. This is when I saw Mr Y. He wrote that I was paranoid—*because I did not like being lied to*. He wrote that I was manipulative and sociopathic—*because I wanted to make decisions about my own treatment*. He wrote of evidence of sexual fetishism—*because I resent having someone else's grotesque aesthetic preferences carved into my penis*. He stuck to their obviously futile and counterproductive plan of ganging up on me and forcing Dr W. on me. Nonetheless, when I canceled the follow up appointments and refused to see Dr. W, they relented and let me see a Polish doctor who has not been mutilated.

To Dr. W, Dr. X, and Mr. Y:

I am here because, *in point of fact*, I was sexually assaulted *by a doctor* and I have feelings about that. He strapped me down—that is bondage. He sexually diminished me *for life*—that is domination. He inflicted excruciating pain—that is sadism. This is the most extreme form of sexual assault. I have spent years of *my life* undoing, to the extent possible, what he did in minutes. I have feelings about that, and that is why I am here. *Get it through your head.*

It is my life, my penis, my feelings; I'm the subject matter expert. You are ignoramuses. I have studied the historical context—*you have not*. I have studied the medical ethics—*you have not*. I have studied the anatomy and physiology of the prepuce—*you have not*. I have studied the resulting complications—*you have not*. I have first hand experience; I have restored my foreskin—*you have not*. You are not merely ignorant. You are willfully ignorant and impervious to new information.

Has it entered your mind for a moment that you are *so dismissive* due to denial about your own disfigured dick? Heaven forbid you should wake up and see the scar on your own mutilated member. Perhaps you're too preoccupied protecting your perception of *your penis* to help your patient?

I have been incredibly patient with you. I have made my case clearly and calmly. I have explained why this is—*in point of fact*—a sexual assault. I have presented evidence that genital mutilation *is not trivial*. You have not made your case. You *merely assert* that it not sexual assault. You have not refuted a single thing that I've said. You have not presented a single shred of evidence. You merely reiterate rationalizations—which you yourself admit are invalid.

It is my life, my penis, my feelings; I am the subject matter expert. I am the one that walks out that door with the outcome of the treatment. I own it. It is my treatment plan. Your role is to facilitate and advise me on *my treatment plan.* It is not your place to force your plan, your goals, your aspirations on me. I am here because a doctor did that to me. It is that approach to medicine, that heady combination of arrogance and ignorance that my assailant carved into my penis.

You have no empathy, no respect and no insight. Your judgment is impaired, and your incompetence is causing iatrogenic rage—*this is what you are treating with those pills.* You want to work it out? I loath and despise you. What is your plan? Are you Peter Pan—will you enchant me with magic pixie dust? You still want to work it out—*you are delusional.* Work this out: I loath and despise you—*our relationship is over!*

Thomas
38 years
Florida, USA
6 April 2014

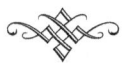

Things Could So Easily Have Been Different

I was born in mid-1947 and circumcised some time in mid-1948. This was in Northern Ireland, part of the United Kingdom (UK). My father was from England and my mother was from here.

Circumcision was, and still is, very rare here. I learned at about age five or six that I was "different." We lived at the seaside, there was frequent swimming with other boys, and it very soon was obvious that it was me who was different. I remember asking my mother about it. All she said was to not show it to anyone. That was the start of my embarrassment and dislike about having been circumcised.

I'm a thin and active person. I like sports but changing for sports, along with showering after, was a bit of a nightmare for me. I used to hide myself whenever I could. To be honest, I don't remember any bad comments being made to me and I'm sure that my attempts to hide were not always one hundred percent successful. I think that if I had been bullied or laughed at because of my circumcised penis, the effect would have been devastating on me.

One other occasion on which I asked my mother about it probably shines some light on the background to the circumcision. My question was answered with: "It's good enough for Prince Charles, so it should be good enough for you." My mother's family were Ulster loyalists. They near worshiped the UK royals. Charles is just a few months younger than I am and it was publicly announced that he had been circumcised. It appears that circumcision is practiced by the UK upper classes and UK royalty.[172] I should say here that we are far from upper class—indeed, at the other extreme!

A further factor was that the UK National Health Service (NHS) had just been set up. Neonatal circumcision was free on parental demand. My parents were relatively poor and I doubt if I would have been circumcised if they had had to pay for it. This situation did not persist for long. Douglas Gairdner's paper "The Fate of the Foreskin"[173] put an end to free-on-demand circumcision in the UK. My parents may have demanded that I be circumcised but it was a "doctor" who took a knife to my penis. I have a

---

[172] For an analysis of the British Royal Family's connection with circumcision see Robert Darby and John Cozijn, "The British Royal Family's Circumcision Tradition,"*SAGE* 3, 4 (2013), accessed 24 December 2013, doi: 10.1177/2158244013508960.

[173] D. Gairdner, "The fate of the foreskin: a study of circumcision," *BMJ* 2 (1949): 1433-7.

continuing deep distrust of medical people.

My father was never able to bring himself to talk about it with me. I can only guess what his thoughts were. He was intact. I had no brothers to talk with about it.

The word "circumcision" was very rarely heard, but I cringed and broke into a sweat any time it was said. Even similar sounding words such as "circumscribed" had the same effect on me. In late childhood or early adolescence I read about circumcision. Only the outlines were described in books of that time—there were no graphic details. Even reading these tame non-graphic explanations further horrified me. I dread to think how I may have reacted if I had seen Internet videos of a circumcision being performed. When I watched one such video in about 2000, I was sick on the desk beside the keyboard.

In other ways I was fortunate. The secondary level school (ages 12 - 18) that I attended was in an agricultural area and was small. It was there that I learned about sex from the fellow students. I developed an interest in electronics and mathematics, which was encouraged by the teachers. I realized that it would be better for me to "escape" from home as soon as I could. Just before leaving the school I had offers of three jobs, all in Belfast. I moved away from the family home and never returned. Relations with my parents were on a formal level thereafter.

One of my first personal acts related to my circumcision was to have a couple of tattoos put on my upper arms. This was primarily to indicate that it is my choice about what happens to my body. It had a secondary effect of diverting attention away from my mutilated penis in naked situations.

I was strongly attracted to females. But, because the embarrassment of having been circumcised still weighed heavy on me, I did not make much of an effort to find females. Several found me! Again I was fortunate—I don't remember any of them making bad remarks about the circumcision. Some were curious and I tried as best as I could to explain. I eventually realized that, when the right woman came along, I would have to be totally open about my feelings on circumcision on the very first occasion that we got naked together. This worked well and we are still married.

My hatred of my circumcision continued. I still hid myself in locker room type situations. When the opportunity to restore a foreskin by non-surgical means became available in the early 1990's, I jumped at it. From the start, I felt considerable relief in being able to correspond with other men who were in a situation similar to myself. Even better was the eventual satisfaction of having a restored foreskin, which is near indistinguishable from the real thing.

I would be pleased to enter into correspondence about any of the above points. T0rm0d@hotmail.com.

Tormod
66 years
Northern Ireland
28 October 2013

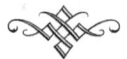

This Barbaric Savage Ritual

This barbaric savage ritual of circumcision was initiated for the first time in Ishtar Temple (Mesopotamia) and Isis Temple (Ancient Egypt). It was a demonic method to produce continuous sexual stimulation by removing the foreskin, the natural protection of the penis.

I was born in Mesopotamia (Iraq today) and I am a victim of MGM.[174] When I was four years old, I was surprised one morning with a big man holding my hands to my back and my father convincing me not to resist! Then I remember they exposed my private organs for people gathered in our house yard. It was public child sexual abuse! Then all I remember is terrible pain and bleeding. For days I was laying naked in bed with wounded and exposed private organs (which seemed not private anymore).

The shock destroyed my self-esteem. I was a very good boy and used to listen to my father; therefore, I was wondering why I was punished so terribly? Why?

When I asked a few years later, some people said, "You are born dirty and circumcision is to purify you"!? Imagine for a child who was in my situation: I was daring to ask them if girls are born perfect and I was born dirty! Such conflict inside my brain destroyed trust in people, my dad, and myself.

A month after I lost my foreskin, I felt the friction of the sensitive glans with my clothes and it produced faint pleasure, which was completely new to me. Then I aimed to make this friction with my hands—believe it or not, I started masturbating at the age of four years. It was devastating to my sexual life, because sex to me was linked to violence and pain. Sadomasochism was inevitable.

Then after many years, I learned that the majority of males in the Arab world are sadomasochists. Many other smart boys turned after circumcision to bisexual behaviors. Bisexual behavior is very common in Arabs and Jews, and also in American cities where circumcision rate is high, like in New York. I have read some research about the relation between circumcision and bisexual behavior. In the Arab gender-separation world it turns to homosexual culture.

I cannot establish normal relations with a woman even though I am over 40 years old now. God damn that barbaric sexual abuse!

---

[174] MGM is male genital mutilation.

I can go longer in my story, telling of more grief and pain and a useless fight against a community that believes in this stupid rite. The worst thing is that if I fight in public against MGM then I would be considered as an "infidel" and sentenced to death by my people.

Circumcision is a curse here in the Middle East. Every June I see mass massacres when millions of boys undergo circumcision in mass parties. It is an unbelievably disgusting scene, with the boys screaming and trying to get themselves loose from old men's hands. The worst that happens is when parents themselves have tied their boy for the butcher. This is a scene of mentally and emotionally sick people, mass madness, the smell of blood, and pale, exhausted victims in shock and trauma. And at the same time, you adults are dancing in a hysteric way, celebrating the pain and humiliation of minors.

This is a completely sick society. I am not surprised after that to see any kind of abnormal behaviors in my community, because I have seen the ultimate shit celebrated in joy.

When I grew up, I discovered that it is impossible with normal intercourse to satisfy my desire. Then I found I lost 20,000 nerve pleasure receptors when I lost my foreskin. Most men in the Arab world try to have many intercourses in one night to get satisfaction equal to one normal intercourse. The inevitable result is frustration and exhaustion. The frustration bursts into violence and even beheading. This crazy society lives obsessed with sex and violence.

I can go on more and more for days, but this is enough because I cannot bear to expose more pain. Just to see the iceberg tip is enough to estimate what is under the water surface.

Muslim Man
43 years
Iraq
11 January 2014

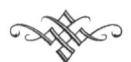

Tricked

First of all, it is extremely difficult for me to write this. Foreskin is a taboo topic for me because the pain and anger it incurs in my heart is too much for me to bear. But for some reason, I was dragged into this topic tonight and it snowballed into outright fury and a need to seek comfort.

To tell the truth, now that I am in my early twenties, I fully understand the magnitude of the mutilation that was done to me and the obscenely dishonest and malicious circumstances by which it was imposed on me when I was barely fourteen.

I have been told SO many lies—so many lies why I should have my prepuce cut or else. They told me it was a medical danger, that if I don't get cut. … I will not be able to have sex at all. I can't have children; no girl will ever want to look at me naked.

They told me it was unhygienic to have a foreskin, that it will be impossible to keep yourself clean, that over time you would develop infection because of the foreskin, and your penis might end up being cut off. They said it was "excess" skin and that it was a mistake of God. That nature got the human body right EXCEPT the foreskin and it needed to be cut or else.

All of these came from my mother. They came from my father. They fed these insane lies to me when I was just twelve to thirteen. What was I supposed to do? How was I supposed to know better?

I feel so violated. I don't know anymore. It is such a cheat. I was so incredibly tricked.

I feel so angry now because I know I was robbed of a fulfilling sex life. I have done my research, and discovered the ONLY reason the foreskin is cut is because ancient people wanted GOD more than they wanted physical sensation. These dark-age bastards have spread the disease of circumcision to pervert us all, to make us less than human, and to make us as psychopathic as them.

I feel so depressed. I want my foreskin back. I remember as a kid I couldn't even pull my skin down,[175] even in the showers. I would jump from the intensity of the sensation, unable to explain how pleasurable it was. In the thirteen years I had my foreskin I had not once been able to pull the skin down. I didn't even know the cock was shaped like a helmet until they cut me. And whenever I would masturbate, it would be slow and sensuous. My

---

[175] "Pulling the skin down" means retracting the foreskin.

mind would be positively swimming.

When they did mutilate me. God. It felt like I didn't have a dick anymore. Before I would use my whole hand to masturbate, but now I can only use my index finger and thumb on a one-inch area of the shaft because the head is now bare. It doesn't feel anything at all! I can remember that when I still had my foreskin it was the HEAD that made me cum. Now, the head is as good as cut off. What good is it if you can't feel anything from it?

I would trade all the cums I have made in the ten years I have been cut in exchange for ONE cum from when I still had my foreskin. To this day, my most memorable sexual experience is me lazily toying with my still intact dick while I was still eleven years old. No experience in my whole teenage years can compare to the pleasure of nonchalantly rubbing my foreskin together. I can never forget the feeling.

I don't know anymore. The more I think about it the more I want to get hit by a bus. This is not the life nature intended for me. I have been tricked when I was still a minor. Mutilated by dozens of lies by my own parents, before I could make a righteous judgment. I can just see those Old Testament saints who started this barbaric practice in the first place laughing at me from their graves. They have victimized me after their deaths!

I know many of you have gone through the same thing. And I'm sure you can relate with the emotional anger and severe depression I am having right now. We have all been cheated. We have all been mutilated. We cannot get back what they took from us.

Chester
24 years
Philippines
4 October 2013

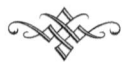

Two Day Old Infant

Two day old infant
It is not yet a person
Have your way with it.

Two day old infant
You decide that you own it
Have your way with it.

Two day old infant
Own it, mark it, brand your thing
Have your way with it.

Two day old infant
Help yourself to its penis
Have your way with it.

Two day old infant
When does it become a him?
What will he think then?

Thomas
38 years
Florida,USA
6 April 2014

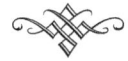

Unnecessary Surgery Ruined My Sex Life

I'm a guy in my thirties who was circumcised for 'phimosis' when I was fourteen in the Perth Royal Infirmary, Scotland.[176]

Neither my parents nor I gave informed consent, because we were never told that it was going to destroy all sensitivity in my penis and consequently ruin my sex life. Also, I have since found out that circumcision is not necessary for phimosis, as stretching can resolve the problem. In those days, we didn't have the World Wide Web, so I really can't blame my parents. I blame the doctor who told me to get it done. The heinous surgeon killed my spirit and, thus, my body and mind when he cut off part of my genitals.

This has caused me devastation throughout my life. As I'm in the UK, this happened on the National Health Service (NHS). I tried to sue the NHS for medical negligence when I was twenty-one, but they told me that there was a time limitation of three years for claims. It's ruined my life: relationships haven't worked, sex has been awkward for the most part due to no feeling, I can't orgasm most of the time during sex due to a complete absence of a frenulum, and it's affected my entire psychology.

So I now find myself jobless and suicidal at the age of thirty-four. I'm at my lowest ebb now, having been thinking of suicide for the past year.

My parents, who are separated now, don't want to know. Firstly, there's nothing they can do, because the problem is irreversible. Secondly, I just don't think they see it as a big deal. And, finally, I think they think I'm exaggerating due to there being other circumcised guys who don't complain. As we all know, you can't take my experience and extrapolate it to every single circumcised guy in the world, because not all circumcisions are created equal; many guys have a lot of their frenulum, so it isn't anywhere near as bad, and restoring is a worthwhile endeavor for them.

I researched foreskin restoration and bought a TLC Tugger.[177] However, after more research, the futility of this seemed obvious to me. With no frenulum (the most sensitive part of the penis) and thus no ejaculatory trigger, what's the point? The glans isn't a very sensitive part of the penis; it detects heat,

---

[176] *Phimosis* is a condition in which the foreskin cannot be retracted. This is perfectly normal in boys. Natural masturbation helps to stretch the skin. In rare pathological situations topical steroids can be used and surgical intervention as a last resort.

[177] TLC Tugger is a foreskin restoration device made by TLCTugger.com.

cold and pain, but isn't a fine touch receptor.[178]

I remember that when I was thirteen or fourteen and began playing with myself, I was able to make myself ejaculate very quickly without being able to retract my foreskin. I also remember an ice cream headache sometimes from masturbating because the feelings were so good. Now when I masturbate, I feel nothing. What I have to do is knead very hard on the point where the frenulum used to be. This allows me to ejaculate eventually, but it's a means to an end and gives me no pleasure. It's just a biological necessity like going to the toilet. I've never felt the glans was a sensitive structure. I've never been able to enjoy sex because all my frenulum and frenulum delta have been ablated.

As I said, this isn't something that has just entered my mind recently. I've been depressed about it since I had it done. It really caused me great anxiety during my twenties and caused lots of awkward situations due to erectile problems. If you can't feel anything, it's difficult to keep it up. When you get your first blow job and you feel nothing, that's frightening. And when you sleep with your first girl but you don't know if you're inside her due to no sensitivity, it drives one insane.

I feel that even people who are aware of the damage circumcision causes tend to downplay just how devastating this can be. It is exactly the same as female genital mutilation, and I simply cannot believe this is still being done legally. Whenever I switch on the television, feminists in the UK are whining about a couple of cases of illegal FGM.[179] Yet everyone ignores the fact that the NHS is still doing MGM[180] on the public purse, for religious reasons and for 'medical' reasons, even though circumcision is rarely medically justifiable.

As for not working, I'm actually in a state of mind now in which I don't want to work. I'm currently at university as a mature student. I'm halfway through a science degree, due to go back tomorrow for the first day of third year, but I'm planning on ordering chloroform when my student loan comes through. I just see no value in life now, so death seems like the only rational solution. I don't want kids and I'm not overly ambitious. All I ever wanted was a comfortable life and to find a nice girl.

---

[178] It is true that most of the glans only detects heat, cold and pain. However, the glans corona does contain some Meissner's corpuscles and after restoration appears to recover a considerable amount of fine touch reception.
[179] FGM is female genital mutilation.
[180] MGM is male genital mutilation.

I realize people are in an impossible situation talking to me. The problem I have with talking to a medical professional is that it's those so-called experts who caused my problem to begin with. I simply can't see how talking to someone paid by the very institution which mutilated me will help, because I'm going to be talking about how their barbarism caused these problems. Given that they won't apologize or compensate me; that they still mutilate boys on the NHS; that they will just shrug their shoulders at the physical damage they caused me, I could see myself going postal on them.[181]

I went to see a urologist when I was twenty-one about this. He just shrugged his shoulders and said, "There may be nerve damage but you can't prove it." I learned afterwards that it's already been established, since chopping off erogenous tissue will result in loss of nerves. I even had one doctor shrug and say, "Well at least you can last longer." Can you imagine the outcry if he'd said that to a female victim of genital mutilation?

Not being able to enjoy sex at all is just crippling for me, especially since I learned of the science behind the working of the penis and why I can't feel anything down there. I actually think MGM is worse than FGM in a way, because there's so much pressure on men. A woman can lie back and not have to do any work; a man has to do all the thrusting. Trying to have sex with a girl in the missionary position when you feel absolutely nothing is just a horrible situation. It's impossible for me to even ejaculate. The only positions I've ever been able to ejaculate were doggy and spooning: it's something to do with friction on the frenulum and the ability to tighten my muscles and concentrate.

The frenular area is the only part of my penis where I can feel anything, and it's only a light tingling, which subsides after a while. I know how sensitive it must have been from when I played with myself before the circumcision. I remember the tingling sensations and how easy it was to orgasm, and that was without retraction. I've never experienced sexual satisfaction since the very day I was circumcised. I've always intuitively known from the horrific moment that I saw the result of my operation that the frenulum was the source of all the pleasure and it had been ablated.

If the NHS in the UK had given me compensation, as I rightly should have received, then maybe I could have sleepwalked through this drudgery for another few decades with the security the money provided. As it stands, I just don't have the enthusiasm, motivation, determination, and hope necessary to keep going. I know I'll never work again. It was a miracle I attended university yesterday, but all I could do was think constantly of

---

[181] *Going postal* is pulling out a firearm and going berserk.

suicide and my circumcision throughout the lectures. It was torture. To top it off, I'm putting on loads and loads of weight, because I just don't have any energy or any motivation to lose weight. What's the point? Lose weight to look good so I can get a woman to have sex with and never be able to feel it?

There's a woman I'm very uneasy even talking to, because ultimately, I will never be able to experience sex in the way that normal, intact people can. I'm constantly thinking about this concept. When I watch films and I see men and women having spontaneous sex, I get anxious and depressed. The fact that I can't feel sex makes the whole courtship and relationship dynamics pointless. Life is sex. Women, more now than ever, demand high standards where sex is concerned.

I don't buy the whole sex in the brain theory. That's fine as an added bonus if you have your full equipment intact and you can achieve sexual satisfaction of the erogenous zones, but for me, without that, it can't act as a substitute. I'm not really someone who has any weird fantasies. I like good-looking women with good bodies and nice personalities; I'm pretty straightforward and uncomplicated. I really can't see me ever finding the motivation and enthusiasm necessary to go out and get a girlfriend ever again. I just avoid women now, as I just don't see any point.

Lawrence
34 years
Perth, Scotland
18 September 2013

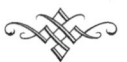

Way To Go, "Doctor"

I was circumcised at birth with a Plastibell.[182] If I could, I would go back eighteen years and find the guy who cut my foreskin off and knee him in the balls for being such a colossal buzzkill.

Wednesday night I was hanging out with my girlfriend. We were in my car, parked in some dark corner somewhere, and things were getting pretty "hot and heavy" as they say. After a while, she pulls back and gives me a funny look, and then works up the courage and offers me a blow/hand job (it was adorable). I put on a cool facade, all like "yeah, sure, that'd be cool I guess" but on the inside I was screaming "AWWEEEESOME!" Now, applying to college and a lot of school nonsense has kind of put my restoring activities on hold, so there was very little slack to work with at this point.

She decides to start with her dry, unlubricated hands.

At this point you're probably all screaming "NO! DON'T DO IT" like you do at the guy who goes alone into the basement to examine the circuit breaker in a horror movie. *It felt like having sex with fire.* I tried to make it work, but I couldn't, so I told her it was too dry, she should try something else. Well, because of the intense friction, I somehow managed to go completely numb (which is better than feeling pain, I guess). She starts to use her mouth and I CAN HARDLY FEEL A THING. Then, after a while, she goes back to using her hands, which feels okay, except the friction seems a little intense since her saliva was the only lubricant.

Well, it took me an HOUR of awkward/semi-painful effort to finally climax. She was so exhausted by the end, God bless her for staying with it; I love her to death for trying. All the while she kept asking what she was doing wrong, and why it was taking so long. I feel so bad for her because she won't accept that it wasn't her fault. To top it all off, I got back home that night, and looked down at my member (which I hadn't been able to see clearly in the darkened car) to find that I have MASSIVE, COMPLETELY DESENSITIZED SORES on my inner foreskin, just below the corona.

---

[182] The Plastibell is a circumcision device invented by Hollister Inc in 1950, consisting of a clear plastic ring with a deep circumferential groove.

My wang is raw and beat up, and my girlfriend feels like a failure (and has really tired arms). Awesome, indeed. To the "doctor" who did this, I'd just like to say: way to go, you ass, you totally ruined my first sexual-type experience.

I need to get back to restoring, or at least get her some lotion.

DPX1
18 years
Minnesota, USA
25 April 2009

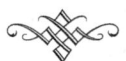

Wounded But Not Broken

I've been aware of my circumcision status since I was a young child, when I first discovered I was born with parts I no longer possess. This occurred after asking my mother for an explanation regarding the distinct brown scar which encircles the shaft of my penis.

She explained to me that I had been circumcised, that men are born with an "unnecessary flap of skin that holds in dirt" on the end of their penis, and that all civilized people have this cut off immediately following birth. This never seemed quite right to me.

Around the age of sixteen I started wearing boxer-briefs rather than briefs because friends had teased me for wearing "tighty-whiteys," as if that were an important social matter. My dick had always stayed securely cradled in the elastic of my underwear with the glans held against my stomach; bizarre, perhaps, but it had allowed the mucosa to remain vibrant pink in color and very sensitive to tactile stimulation.

After switching to loose underwear, I dealt with the discomfort and pain of my dick swinging around and scraping against fabric all day. Eventually the pain and discomfort subsided. I also started washing the actual glans and inner foreskin remnant with soap, when a friend said that he was shocked I did not. I never had directly washed the mucosa of my penis, which I know now was wise. The mucous membrane of the genitalia, like any other, is meant to be very thin and always a bit moist. But after so much exposure to the drying and roughening effects of unnatural exposure to air, abrasion, and soap, my mucous membrane had become brown, leathery, and completely insensitive.

At this point, I was distressed, yet still sane. I was doing research one night on male sexuality, totally unrelated to my issue, and came across information regarding circumcision. As my eyes darted around the screen in shock and revolted awe, I felt a flood of agony engulf me. I was completely sexually numb, at seventeen. To make matters worse, I was in the midst of my first romantic love affair.

I was spiritually shattered, I had no defense; I suffer from a non-operational denial mechanism. I simply can't lie to myself. I crawled into the walk-in closet, as I lived with family and had nowhere else to hide. I sobbed and felt my skin crawling all over my body, the vivid sensation of knives stabbing into my heart and abdomen. I recall feeling as if malevolent, unseen entities were tearing at my flesh, consuming me alive.

How could this happen in these United States, in 1983? Somebody tied me down, put me through the worst physical agony imaginable, and left me scarred and missing most of my sexual nerve endings. And now I was COMPLETELY numb. I freaked out on my partner, who was intact; my jealousy was unbearable. What had he done to be spared? He was born premature, to an old Italian doctor in Upstate New York in 1961, that's what. It was simply a matter of good fortune, or in my case, the lack thereof. It was all about the luck of the draw.

The emotional pain was so intense that every night I would pray that I would not awake again the next morning. I started self-mutilating by burning myself with cigarettes, and often using psychoactive substances to obliterate all consciousness to try and escape the agony. Eventually I was forced into a mental health crisis unit for suicidal ideation.

Once there, I told the intake people why I was breaking down. I was utterly cognizant and I explained myself articulately, despite being suicidally depressed. The intake nurse told me "But every man in the world is circumcised." I informed her of the reality regarding that. "Well, my husband is circumcised and he's never had any problems." Oh, my dear, if you and he only knew, I thought to myself.

I was delusional in their eyes. I know that's what went into the charts. The next day, I saw a psychiatrist. I gave him my self-diagnosis of Bi-Polar II, which I came to from Internet research. In reality I also have Borderline Personality Disorder—which was exacerbated by this sexual trauma. The psychiatrist asked me if I had ever had any major surgeries other than my circumcision. He had a smirk on his face when he mentioned the circumcision aspect.

I was seventeen and he looked to be in his mid-twenties at the oldest. The audacity on his part, to assume I must be completely stupid and oblivious even to his obvious grin of superiority as he placated me; that I must be stupid and delusional to think circumcision was harmful in any way. Needless to say, that was not the kind of help I required.

I was given serotonin reuptake inhibitors and mood stabilizers, which helped bring my acute agony down to a simmering, throbbing, sorrowful rage. I was employed at a nursing home full-time, and highly valued the emotional connections I made with the residents. I clung to my boyfriend for security, drank a lot of alcohol, and tried my best to avoid thoughts about my mutilation.

I did some restoration exercises at that time in my life, primarily via the "T-Tape Method," which loosened the skin enough to allow me to apply a tape-ring around the skin pulled to the fore of my glans, to keep my shaft skin forward all the time and therefore protect the mucous membrane of my genitalia from direct exposure. This allowed me to shed a massive amount of keratin. The layers of keratin form a callous which numbs the remaining inner foreskin of a circumcised penis.[183] As the keratin sloughed away, I regained a lot of sexual sensitivity and my mucosa became bright pink and supple. I became lazy and made no attempts at restoration for years, always keeping my penis wrapped up by its tape-ring when I wasn't urinating or engaged in sexual activity.

I wanted to sue the doctor who mutilated me, but I had passed the Florida statute of limitations, as I was too traumatized to bring myself to see a lawyer when I was still eighteen. The doctor who had cut me is dead anyway. My mother has apologized for what happened, and she feels guilty. I've told her in recent times not to feel guilty, because I know she didn't know any better. But I admit I feel like I wasn't protected. Deep down I often feel as if there is no security in this world.

I spent most of my twenties in a drugged haze, trying to avoid the pain of my mutilation, as well as other traumas I experienced throughout my childhood and adolescence. My mutilation drove me to the verge of suicide many times. I am in no way implying that most men who realize the negative impact of their circumcisions become this distraught. However, I have spoken to many others who have been just as badly damaged emotionally and psychologically by the mutilation as I am, and some who feel even considerably worse.

During my wild teens and twenties, I was highly promiscuous. I have met many men who feel nothing or barely anything during sex. I have also been with many intact men, and also many circumcised men who feel varying amounts of pleasure from sexual stimulation. From extensive research and experience, working in unison, I have developed a comprehensive, lucid understanding of male genital anatomy and sexual experience which transcends that of everyone I know other than a few individuals who are also unhappily circumcised gay men.

---

[183] It is a common belief that the glans surface (mucosa) becomes more thickened (keratinized) as a result of circumcision. One study found no difference, see Dinh M.H. et al. "Keratinization of the adult male foreskin and implications for male circumcision" *AIDS* 24, 6 (2010): 899-906.

The glans of the penis is not the focal point for sexual pleasure for most intact or even most cut men. The frenular delta is the seat of male sexual pleasure: it is the "male clitoris." The glans is not. The glans is innervated with nerve endings which primarily record sensations of pain, pressure and changes in temperature. Meissner's corpuscles are the fine-touch nerve endings responsible for the most intense sensations of sexual pleasure. They are found in only small quantities spread thinly across the glans, with somewhat higher concentrations in the corona (the ridge) and near the tip just above the urethra. The glans can indeed feel significant pleasure, but it mainly provides a supportive type of sensation to the fine-touch ecstasy of the frenular delta.

The frenulum connects the glans to the foreskin and shaft in a manner that causes the foreskin to remain forward when not intentionally retracted. It looks and functions similarly to the frenulum under the tongue. The ridged band, which is heavily innervated with Meissner's corpuscles, is composed of tight ridges of mucosa.

These areas all converge to create the frenular delta, which is an inch or so below the glans on an intact penis when the foreskin is fully retracted. Some circumcised men have a significant portion of the ridged band left, and therefore feel significant sexual pleasure. Others have none of those tissues remaining, and are left with only the glans for stimulation.

For me, stimulation of the glans without stimulation of the frenular delta is uncomfortable and can even be painful; my glans only feels pleasure when stimulated in conjunction with the frenular area below it. Other men feel more pleasure from glans stimulation alone. However, all men I've encountered who still have frenular areas which give pleasure find the latter much more important to their sexual enjoyment.

When a boy is circumcised, it is impossible to know just how much sexual pleasure he will be left with. My soul-mate was circumcised so loosely that he functions more like an intact man than a circumcised one. He was cut via the Mogen Clamp.[184] This clamp often results in very loose circumcisions, and especially spares the frenular area due to its design. It has been taken off the market, after a class action lawsuit, as many babies had their entire glans amputated due to the specific nature of the device.

---

[184] The Mogen Clamp is a circumcision device invented by Rabbi Harry Bronstein in 1954.

My soul-mate has all of his frenular delta left intact, and has full glans coverage when flaccid and partial when erect. This is very rare, and he is very fortunate. But if the doctor had taken just a millimeter more frenular flesh through the clamp before bearing-down, he would have lost part of the delta and therefore would feel considerably less sexually than he fortunately does. And, of course, it was still agonizing for him when it happened as a defenseless infant, and it could have meant his life.

At least 100 babies are reported to die from circumcision complications annually in the United States alone.[185] And remember, there are certainly deaths which are not attributed publicly to circumcision but which were in truth caused by such. The knowledge base of developmental psychology makes it obvious that such intense pain experienced at that young age also has long-term psychological ramifications.

I could go on forever about this topic, as the ramifications are just so very colossal, so deep and wide that I can't even comprehend all of it. We are the only first-world nation which does this to our infants en masse. To fight against female genital mutilation in Africa whilst recommending mass circumcisions of men all over the world is insanely provincial and misguided.

Like it or not, sex is an extremely important component of human experience. For the most part, it is a beautiful thing. Our sexual organs and brain chemistry make it possible for us to experience heights of sexual pleasure unlike any other organism on Earth. This occurs both to make life beautiful for each and every one of us, as well as to bind us to one another. To give exquisite pleasure to a person one loves deeply is the most beautiful thing in the world.

All forms of sexual mutilation succeed in further complicating an already complicated matter, that of communicating and bonding with another via sexual activity. Maimonides, the medieval Jewish philosopher, said outright in his writings that circumcision is intended to drastically reduce sexual pleasure. He said:

> Similarly with regard to circumcision, one of the reasons for it is, in my opinion, the wish to bring about a decrease in sexual intercourse and a weakening of the organ in question, so that this activity be diminished and the organ be in as quiet a state as possible. It has been thought that

---

[185] It is estimated that 117 circumcision deaths occur annually in the US. This represents 1.3% of all neonatal male deaths from all causes. Dan Bollinger, "Lost boys: An estimate of U.S. circumcision-related infant deaths," *Thymos: Journal of Boyhood Studies* 4, 1 (2010): 78-90.

circumcision perfects what is defective congenitally. This gave the possibility to everyone to raise an objection and to say: How can natural things be defective so that they need to be perfected from outside, all the more because we know how useful the foreskin is for that member? In fact this commandment has not been prescribed with a view to perfecting what is defective congenitally, but to perfecting what is defective morally. The bodily pain caused to that member is the real purpose of circumcision. None of the activities necessary for the preservation of the individual is harmed thereby, nor is procreation rendered impossible, but violent concupiscence and lust that goes beyond what is needed are diminished. The fact that circumcision weakens the faculty of sexual excitement and sometimes perhaps diminishes the pleasure is indubitable. For if at birth this member has been made to bleed and has had its covering taken away from it, it must indubitably be weakened. The Sages, may their memory be blessed, have explicitly stated: It is hard for a woman with whom an uncircumcised man has had sexual intercourse to separate from him. In my opinion this is the strongest of the reasons for circumcision.[186]

Is this what you want for your children? How can something stolen be said to be a willing sacrifice? If a man truly wants to prove his allegiance to his God by giving up his most sexually pleasurable body parts, won't his conviction be all the more clearer by him making this decision as an informed adult, and going through the experience with intent, precision, and spiritual meaning?

We do not allow Muslims, some of whom choose to cut both boy and girl genitals, to do so to their female offspring, by threat of law. Yet males remain unprotected.

Today, I am once again actively restoring my foreskin, using devices I've obtained from innovative and caring intactivists who sell their devices for the benefit of all of us. I have enough flesh down there to cover my glans when flaccid without the help of tape. Erect coverage will not come as easily, due to the large size of my member and the fact that I was cut very tightly. But

---

[186] Moses Maimonides, *The Guide Of The Perplexed*, p.609, http://www.cirp.org/library/cultural/maimonides/ (accessed 1 January 2014). Without a knowledge of sex hormones Maimonides aligns himself with the ancients in ascribing the sex drive to the anatomy. (The late nineteenth and early twentieth century clergy and physicians fell into the same fallacy in their misandrist drive to tone down male sexuality.) He also ascribes a "life-force" to the blood, another very ancient concept. Maimonides completely ignores the increased level of male sexual frustration that arises from being deprived of the normal penile sensory input that the brain expects.

the amount of sexual pleasure I am now able to experience is far higher than what I felt before beginning restoration. I recommend it to all cut men.

I was cut via the Plastibell and, like most who had that method, have a good amount of inner foreskin left, but the sensation is uneven, as is the scar-line. In the left ventral (bottom) area, in my frenular-delta remnant, there is intense pleasurable sensation. I lost all the flesh that would have originally been the outer penile shaft and foreskin, it now being migrated pubic-mound skin that is hairy, which grows to the scar-line. After all, can someone draw a dotted-line where the foreskin ends and the "true penis" begins? There is no dotted-line because there is no clear differentiation. Like the finger that is part of the hand as well as its own entity, the foreskin is an integral part of the mammalian penis. It evolved into the highly complex and beautifully functional state it currently holds for a reason. There is no dilemma when one is birthing a baby boy of whether or not to circumcise him. The answer should be clear as day to anyone with all the information and healthy motives.

And remember, never retract a child's foreskin forcibly. I've seen so much damage in the US from the few fortunate intact men of my generation and the couple of generations preceding mine, from foolish and ignorant "exploration" of the inside of the penis during their childhoods. There are texts that explain all this exhaustively, I recommend looking at *Mothering.com* for one, for any prospective parent of a newborn boy.

It is obvious to me that the jealousy so many circumcised men feel for intact men is the main motivator in continuing the mutilation in many instances. Take for example the American Academy of Pediatrics, which is run almost completely by circumcised men. In the face of overwhelming evidence that circumcision has no benefits at all and the evidence of how amazingly wonderful the foreskin really is, they still maintain that circumcision has some benefits and that it should be the parents' choice to have it done if they wish.

Yet we don't allow other body parts to be cut off of infants for so-called prophylactic medical care. Why, there are many body parts that are much less useful and far more likely to be problematic than the foreskin. Why no preventative mastectomies, fingernail removal, etc? Could it be that people are not applying logic to the topic of circumcision whatsoever?

Me, I will survive, and I will thrive as far as that is possible; I will not allow myself to be defeated by this awful practice. But the scars will always be there, both the ones on my penis and the ones on my psyche and soul. I still cry myself to sleep some nights, the hideous screams of a baby boy in the midst of mutilation filling my ears. Only through activism do I find a modicum of psychological comfort.

Let's spare our future generations, shall we?

Jaime Banks
30 years
Pennsylvania, USA
31 December 2013

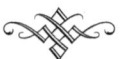

Glossary

CAT Constant Applied Tension, a foreskin restoration device available from www.catstretcher.com.

Circumcision Coma The state of mind of a circumcised person typified by denial that they have been harmed anatomically, physiologically, and psychologically.

Circumstraint A plastic molded board used to immobilize infants for procedures such as circumcision, manufactured by the Olympic Medical Company, Seattle, WA.

Coverage Index A classification system that gives numerical values to describe the length of a foreskin. See: http://www.newforeskin.biz/.

Dartos muscle A layer of smooth muscle within the penile and scrotal skin that contracts in response to low temperatures.

DTR Dual Tension Restorer sold by www.foreskinrestore.com.

Foregen A non-profit organization established to promote the development of regenerative tissue technology in the hope of providing circumcised men with a replacement foreskin.

FGM Female genital mutilation

Frenectomy Surgical removal of the frenulum.

Frenular Delta An erogenous, triangular area of highly sensitive inner foreskin mucosa on the underside side of the penis, centred on the *frenulum,* bounded by the *ridged band* and the *junctional zone,* and richly endowed with *Meissner's corpuscles.*

Frenulum An erogenous web of skin that connects the underside of the glans to the foreskin's *ridged band*, which returns the retracted foreskin over the glans and which tends to control the length of penile strokes during intercourse.

Glans The relatively insensitive, rounded head of the penis that is usually covered by the foreskin.

Glossary

Gomco Clamp A circumcision device developed by Hiram S. ("Inch") Yellen and Aaron A. Goldstein and used in the USA from 1935.

Hematoma (Bruise) A local accumulation of blood leaked from the blood vessels.

Intact (Penis) A natural penis complete with foreskin.

Intactivism The movement promoting genital integrity for all children: male, female and intersex.

Junctional Zone The place at the end of the flaccid foreskin where the outer skin and inner mucosa meet.

Malapposition The misalignment of two opposing bodily structures.

Meatal Stenosis A narrowing of the opening of the urethra, resulting in a reduced urine flow. Commonly found in circumcised boys.

Meatotomy The process of surgically enlarging the urethral opening.

Meatus Opening of the urethra at the end of the penis.

Meissner Corpuscle A capsule-like structure at the end of a nerve axon that accurately detects fine touch and movement. Found in the foreskin, frenulum, and to a lesser extent in the glans corona.

MGM Male genital mutilation

Mogen Clamp A circumcision device invented by Rabbi Harry Bronstein in 1954.

Mohel A Jewish ritual circumciser.

Mucosa Permanent smooth and moist skin on the inner foreskin and covering the glans of intact males.

NOCIRC The National Organization of Circumcision Information Resource Centers. An educational non-profit organization based in California committed to intactivism.

NORM The National Organization of Restoring Men, founded in San Francisco in 1990.

Penile Uncircumcising Device A foreskin restoration device invented by Roland Clark and patented in 1996.

Penoscrotal Webbing A complication of circumcision in which the skin of the scrotum is connected along underside of the penis for a greater distance than normal.

Phimosis A condition in which the foreskin cannot be retracted.

Plastibell A circumcision device invented by Hollister Inc in 1950, consisting of a clear plastic ring with a deep circumferential groove.

Prepuce Foreskin

PUD See *Penile Uncircumcising Device.*

RIC Routine infant circumcision. Circumcision performed on an infant boy without specific medical indications.

Ridged Band A zone of ridged tissue running from the frenulum, around the inside of the tip of foreskin and back to the frenulum. It lies between the outer skin and the smooth inner mucosa and is the primary erogenous penile tissue. It is heavily endowed with *Meissner's corpuscles* in the peaks of the ridges.

Skin Bridge A bridge of skin between the damaged mucosa and the glans formed during the healing process after circumcision.

Skin Tag A non-functional mass of tissue.

Sulcus The groove around the penile shaft where it meets the *glans.*

Synechium The shared membrane connecting the *glans* to the inside of the foreskin.

TLC Tugger A foreskin restoration device made by TLC Tugger.com.

TLC-X Tugger A tapeless foreskin restoration device invented by Ron Low.

Glossary

TUG-A-HOY A tapeless foreskin restoration device invented by Dr James A. Haughey and patented in 2003.

Your Skin Cone A device manufactured by TLCTugger.com used to keep any remnant foreskin covering the glans to help regain lost sensitivity.

Select Bibliography

Brayton, Jerry, "My circumcision story, as told to J. Steven Svoboda", in Chantal Zabus (ed.), *Fearful Symmetries: Essays and Testimonies around Excision and Circumcision* (Amsterdam and New York: Rodopi, 2009); Online at: http://arclaw.org/sites/default/files/Chantal-Zabus-Fearful-Symmetries.pdf

Bigelow, Jim, *The Joy of Uncircumcising!: Exploring Circumcision: History, Myths, Psychology, Restoration, Sexual Pleasure and Human Rights* (Aptos: Hourglass Publishing, 1992).

Bisque, Lisa, *You Call This Love?* (Lincoln: Writer Club Press, 2000).

Boyd, B. R., *Circumcision: What it Does* (San Francisco: Taterhill Press, 1990).

Darby, Robert J. L., 'The child's right to an open future: is the principle applicable to non-therapeutic circumcision?' *Journal of Medical Ethics* published online January 30, 2013 doi: 10.1136/medethics-2012-101182

Darby, Robert, *The Sorcerer's Apprentice: why can't the United States stop circumcising boys?* (Kindle Edition, SJF Publishing, 2013).

Darby, Robert & Cox, Laurence, "Objections of a sentimental character: The subjective dimension of foreskin loss", in Chantal Zabus (ed.), *Fearful Symmetries: Essays and Testimonies around Excision and Circumcision* (Amsterdam and New York: Rodopi, 2009); online at http://www.circinfo.org/documents/ObjectionsSentimental-Zabus.pdf.

Glick, Leonard B., *Marked in Your Flesh: Circumcision from Ancient Judea to Modern America* (York: Oxford University Press, 2005).

Goldman Ronald, *Circumcision: The Hidden Trauma* (Boston: Vanguard Publications, 1997).

Gollaher, David L., *Circumcision: A History of the World's Most Controversial Surgery* (New York: Basic Books, 2000).

Hammond, T. A., "Preliminary Poll of Men Circumcised in Infancy or Childhood," *British Journal of Urology International* 83, Suppl. 1 (1999): 85-92.

Hammond, T. A., *Global Survey of Circumcision Harm.* Online at: http://www.circumcisionharm.org/results.htm.

O'Hara, Karen & O'Hara, John, *Sex As Nature Intended It* (Hudson: Turning Point, 2002).

Peterson, Shane, "Assaulted and mutilated: A personal account of circumcision trauma", in George C. Denniston, Frederick Hodges and Marilyn Milos (eds), *Understanding circumcision: A multi-disciplinary approach to a multi-dimensional problem*, London and New York, Kluwer Academic and Plenum Press, 2001. Online at: http://www.historyofcircumcision.net/index.php?option=com_content&task=view&id=93&Itemid=50.

Robinett, Patricia, *The Rape of Innocence* (Eugene, Nunzio Press, 2010).

Romberg, Rosemary, *Circumcision: The Painful Dilemma* (Massachusetts: Bergin & Garvey, 1985).

Index

About The Author

Lindsay R. Watson, BScHons, DipTchg, is an independent New Zealand researcher. This book is a product of his researches into the changing attitudes and treatment of male sexuality during the nineteenth and twentieth centuries. He is currently researching the New Zealand history of the social and health issues related to the non-therapeutic circumcision of male minors, from ancient Polynesia to the present. He has also researched the New Zealand sexual purity campaigns of Henry Bligh of the Australasian White Cross League (1902-1930).

Published work:

Lindsay R. Watson, "The Universal Condition: Medical Constructions of 'Congenital Phimosis' in Twentieth Century New Zealand and their Implications for Child Rearing," *Health & History* 16, no. 1 (2014): 87-106.

Lindsay R. Watson, "Tom Tiddler's Ground: Irregular Practitioners and Male Sexual Problems in New Zealand, 1858-1908," *Medical History* 57, no. 4 (2013): 537-558.